Hair Braiding

A Step by Step Guide to Mastering Styles, Techniques, and the Cultural Art of Braiding for All Hair Types

Copyright@2024

Colleen Guido

Purpose of the Book

The purpose of this book is in twofold:

1. Technical Mastery: To guide readers through the path of learning and perfecting various hair braiding techniques, from beginner to advanced styles. The book aims to provide clear, step by step instructions that make it accessible for readers with varying levels of experience. It offers practical knowledge about tools, hair types, and styling methods while addressing common challenges and mistakes.

2. Personal Growth and Empowerment: Beyond learning the craft, the book seeks to humanize the braiding experience by focusing on personal development. It emphasizes how the process of braiding can foster creativity, patience, and self-confidence.

Ultimately, this book combines technical expertise with emotional and psychological growth, making

it not just a guide to braiding but also a tool for
personal empowerment.

Table of Contents

Chapter 1

Introduction to Hair Braiding

Hair braiding is the practice of interweaving strands of hair to create intricate patterns or styles. It's a method of hairstyling that has been used for centuries across various cultures, serving as both a practical and artistic way to manage hair. Braiding can be done on any hair type and length, and the complexity of the styles can range from simple three-strand braids to more advanced techniques like French, Dutch, fishtail, and box braids.

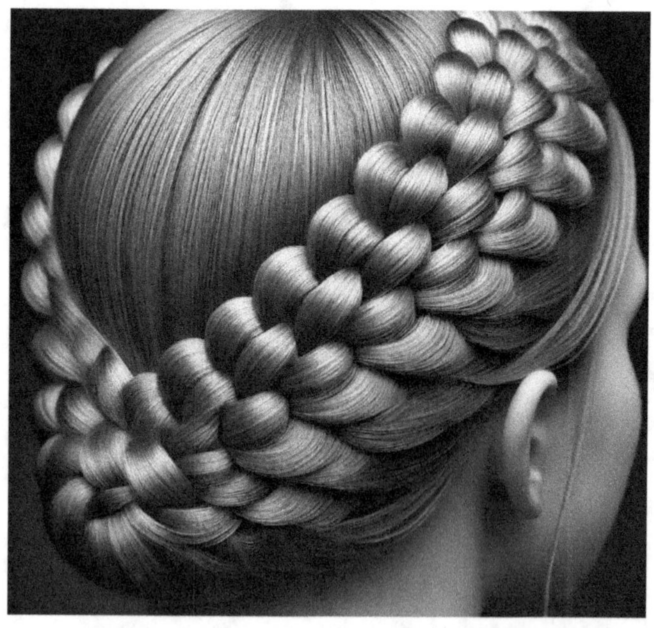

Key Aspects of Hair Braiding:

1. **Interweaving Strands:** At its core, braiding involves dividing hair into sections (typically three or more) and crossing them over each other in a systematic way to create a braid.

2. **Versatility:** Braids can be tight or loose, small or large, depending on the desired style, and can be accessorized with beads, ribbons, or other embellishments.

3. **Cultural Significance:** In many cultures, braiding has deep historical and social meanings. For example, in African communities, different braid patterns can symbolize one's age, marital status, tribe, or wealth.

4. **Practicality:** Braids are often chosen for their protective benefits, as they can keep hair neat and tangle-free for long periods,

minimizing breakage and reducing the need for frequent maintenance.

Types of Hair Braids:

1. Simple Three-Strand Braid: The most basic braid where three strands of hair are alternated by crossing them over each other.

2. French Braid: A more intricate braid that begins at the crown of the head, with new sections of hair added as you work downward.

3. Dutch Braid: Similar to the French braid but with the strands woven under one another, creating a raised, 3D effect.

4. Fishtail Braid: A two-strand braid where small sections of hair are crossed from one side to the other, creating a more delicate, fish-scale-like pattern.

5. Cornrows and Box Braids: Popular in African cultures, these involve tighter braiding patterns that lie flat against the scalp or are individually braided for protective styling.

In addition to aesthetics, hair braiding can serve functional purposes like keeping hair out of the face, protecting hair from environmental damage, and even helping hair retain moisture when done properly with the right care products.

1. History of Hair Braiding

Hair braiding is not just a modern hairstyle but an ancient art form that has transcended cultures, geographies, and eras. From the intricate cornrows of African traditions to the elegant French braids of European aristocracy, braiding has been a means of personal expression, social identity, and cultural heritage. It was often used to indicate status, age, tribe, and even marital status. Today, hair braiding remains a versatile and timeless practice that connects people with both their past and present.

Cultural Significance of Hair Braiding

Hair braiding is more than just a beautiful form of styling it holds deep cultural significance across various societies and time periods. Throughout history, braids have been used as a symbol of identity, tradition, status, and beauty in many cultures around the world. Here are some examples of the cultural importance of braiding:

1. African Culture:

In African cultures, braiding is a centuries-old tradition that carries significant social and cultural meaning. The complexity of a person's braid style often indicated their tribal affiliation, social status, marital status, age, or religious beliefs. Hairstyles like cornrows, box braids, and Fulani braids are still celebrated today for their intricate patterns and protective qualities, while also being a strong connection to African heritage.

Storytelling Through Hair: In some African societies, braiding patterns were a way to tell stories or communicate messages. Braids could symbolize power, wealth, and even convey one's readiness for marriage.

Social Activity: Braiding is often a social activity, where women (and men) gather in groups to braid each other's hair, passing down techniques and cultural traditions through generations.

2. Native American Culture:

For many Native American tribes, hair is considered sacred, and how it is braided holds symbolic meaning. Traditionally, long braids symbolize strength, wisdom, and an individual's connection to the Earth. The practice of braiding hair is a form of reverence and connection to spirituality and nature.

Ceremonial Significance: Braids are worn during important ceremonies, such as weddings and spiritual gatherings. In some tribes, the way a person braids their hair can reflect the tribe they belong to, and their roles in their community.

Warrior Braid: Historically, warriors would braid their hair before battle, as a symbol of readiness and strength.

3. Indian Culture:

In Indian culture, braiding is a common hairstyle among women, especially for formal events or rituals. Long, braided hair is often associated with femininity and spirituality, and is featured prominently in religious and cultural celebrations.

Bridal Braids: During weddings, Indian brides often wear long, elaborately decorated braids, adorned with flowers, gold, or jewels, symbolizing beauty and prosperity.

Hair Oiling and Care: In Indian tradition, hair care rituals like oiling and braiding have been passed down for generations. Oiled braids are a symbol of nurtured and healthy hair, showing a connection between beauty and self-care.

4. Nordic and Celtic Traditions:

In Nordic and Celtic cultures, braids were not only practical but also symbolic. Vikings were known for their elaborate braided hairstyles, which were often used to signify strength and warrior status.

Braided Warriors: Vikings wore their hair in braids to keep it neat during battles. For both men and women, braids were often adorned with beads or rings, symbolizing wealth and prestige.

Celtic Knot Braids: In ancient Celtic traditions, braided patterns reflected nature and life's interconnectedness. Celtic knots and braids were believed to symbolize eternity, with no beginning or end, often used in religious and spiritual contexts.

5. Medieval European Culture:

In medieval Europe, braided hair was a symbol of status and modesty. During this period, long hair was considered a sign of beauty and virtue, and braiding it was a way for women to display their social class.

Intricate Braids for the Elite: The nobility often wore elaborate braided styles to signify their status. Braiding hair was a skill that young girls were taught to demonstrate their femininity and domestic abilities.

Symbol of Modesty: Married women would typically wear their hair braided and covered, as a sign of modesty, while unmarried women often displayed their braids as a sign of their eligibility for marriage.

6. Modern and Contemporary Significance:

Today, braiding continues to be a powerful expression of cultural identity, personal style, and social movements. In particular, braids have seen a resurgence in fashion and media, often reflecting a celebration of natural hair and cultural pride.

Black Hair Movement: In the African American community, braided styles like cornrows and box braids have become symbols of cultural resistance and empowerment. They signify a return to natural hair textures and styles, rejecting historical pressures to conform to Western beauty standards.

Global Popularity: Braids have become a universal hairstyle, popularized in mainstream fashion, from runway models to everyday wear. However, discussions around cultural appropriation have emerged, highlighting the importance of understanding and respecting the cultural origins of braided styles.

2. The Therapeutic Benefits of Braiding

Beyond its cultural significance, hair braiding offers numerous psychological and emotional benefits, acting as a therapeutic activity that promotes mindfulness and stress relief. Braiding requires focus, which can help clear the mind and provide a calming effect. It also nurtures creativity, as the practice involves designing and experimenting with different patterns, textures, and accessories.

Mindfulness and Meditation: The repetitive, rhythmic motion of braiding promotes a mindful state, similar to knitting or drawing, which helps reduce anxiety and promotes mental relaxation.

Stress Relief: Engaging in braiding can help reduce the overwhelm of daily stress, allowing individuals to focus on a task that has a tangible outcome.

Boosting Creativity: Whether experimenting with styles or inventing new techniques, braiding offers limitless possibilities to express one's artistic side.

3. Building Confidence and Self-Esteem Through Braiding

Braiding is more than a hairstyle it's an art form that can empower individuals, build confidence, and boost self-esteem. Whether you're learning to braid for yourself, styling others, or simply experimenting with creative looks, the process of braiding can have a profound impact on how we see ourselves and how we express our identity. Here's how braiding can help you develop confidence and self-esteem through creativity, skill-building, and personal expression.

1. Learning a Skill Boosts Self-Efficacy

Mastering the art of braiding is a tangible skill that requires patience, practice, and dedication. As you develop your braiding skills, you gain a sense of achievement and self-efficacy the belief in your ability to accomplish tasks and overcome challenges.

Celebrating Progress: Whether you're starting with a simple three-strand braid or mastering intricate styles like fishtail or French braids, each step in your braiding journey allows you to measure progress. Over time, as your braids become more polished, you'll build confidence in your skills and abilities.

Overcoming Challenges: Every braid requires focus and coordination, and you may face challenges like uneven sections, loose strands, or mastering tension. Learning to tackle these challenges, problem-solve, and improve with each attempt builds resilience and strengthens your ability to persist through difficulties, which translates into other areas of life.

2. Personal Expression and Individuality

Braiding allows you to express your personal style, culture, and creativity. By experimenting with different braiding techniques, you can shape your outward appearance in a way that reflects who you are. This kind of self-expression helps build a positive relationship with yourself and your identity.

Creative Freedom: Whether you want to try edgy, bold braids or romantic, loose styles, braiding gives you the freedom to experiment with different looks that suit your mood or personality. Expressing yourself through hair allows you to take ownership of how you present yourself to the world, which can help boost self-esteem and reinforce your sense of individuality.

Cultural Pride: For many people, braiding is a way to connect with their cultural roots and traditions. Wearing styles that are symbolic of your heritage or personal history can be a source of pride and confidence, as it allows you to celebrate and share your culture with others.

3. Control Over Your Appearance

One of the most empowering aspects of learning to braid is the sense of control it gives you over your appearance. Styling your own hair, or helping someone else feel beautiful, can be incredibly fulfilling and reinforce positive feelings of self-worth.

Boosting Self-Worth: Braiding allows you to take control of your own grooming and self-care. When you put time and effort into braiding your hair, the final result becomes a reflection of your commitment to yourself. This helps build self-esteem by reminding you that you are worth investing time and care in.

Feeling Accomplished: Whether you're getting ready for a special occasion or simply braiding your hair for the day, completing a braid can give you a sense of accomplishment and confidence in your appearance. Wearing a beautifully styled braid that you created yourself can enhance your self-image and make you feel proud of how you look.

4. Braiding as a Meditative and Mindful Practice

Braiding can also be a meditative practice that brings focus and calm, helping you reconnect with yourself. By practicing braiding regularly, you can reduce stress, increase mindfulness, and boost your overall mental well-being.

Calming Focus: The repetitive motions involved in braiding, such as sectioning, crossing, and weaving strands of hair, can help you stay present and focused on the task at hand. This meditative process is calming, helping your de-stress and quiet your mind, which can lead to increased self-awareness and mental clarity.

Confidence in Mastery: As you become more skilled at braiding, the process becomes smoother and more fluid. This sense of mastery knowing you can create something intricate and beautiful can be deeply satisfying and enhance your confidence, not only in braiding but in other areas of life that require focus and precision.

5. Braiding as a Social Bonding Activity

Braiding has long been a social activity that fosters connection and community, which can also help build confidence and a sense of belonging. Whether you're braiding your own hair or someone else's, it provides an opportunity for positive social interaction, support, and affirmation.

Building Connections: Braiding for family or friends strengthens relationships through shared experiences. The act of braiding someone's hair can be a form of care and affection, deepening emotional bonds. This nurturing act, in turn, builds a sense of community and mutual support.

Receiving Compliments: When others notice and compliment your braiding skills, it boosts your confidence and provides validation of your hard work and creativity. Similarly, complimenting someone else on their braid can uplift them, creating a positive, confidence-building exchange.

6. Overcoming Perfectionism and Embracing Self-Acceptance

Braiding isn't about perfection it's about practice, patience, and self-expression. Learning to accept imperfections in your braids and recognizing the beauty in your progress can help you develop a more compassionate and positive attitude toward yourself.

Letting Go of Perfectionism: No braid is ever perfect, and that's okay. Allow yourself to make mistakes and view them as part of the learning process. As you practice, you'll gain confidence in your ability to improve over time without being weighed down by the pressure to be flawless.

Embracing Your Unique Style: Braiding encourages you to explore different techniques and styles that reflect your individuality. There's no "right" way to braid whether you create loose, messy braids or tight, intricate designs, each braid is a reflection of your personal path and creativity. Learning to appreciate your own unique style can greatly improve your self-esteem.

Braiding is more than just a way to style hair, it's a reflection of history, heritage, and identity. Across cultures, braiding has been used to express social status, tell stories, and create a sense of community. Whether for practical reasons or as a symbol of cultural pride, braiding continues to be an important and cherished tradition that connects us to our roots and allows us to express our individuality.

Chapter 2

Essential Tools for Hair Braiding

To achieve the best results when braiding hair, it's important to use the right tools and products. Whether you're a beginner or more experienced, having these essentials will make the process smoother and help create cleaner, more defined braids. Here's a breakdown of the key tools and their purposes:

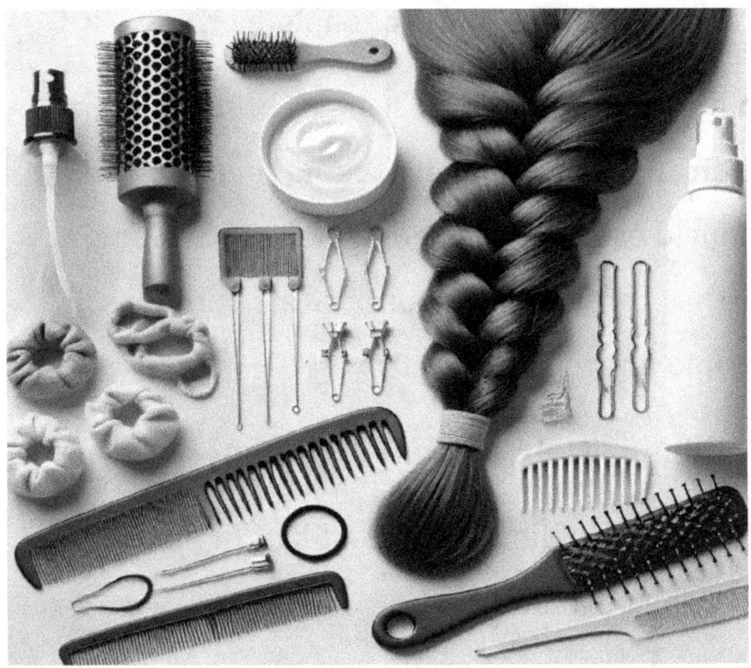

1. Wide Tooth Comb

Purpose: Detangling hair before braiding.

Why It's Important: Hair should be free of tangles and knots to make the braiding process easier and smoother. A wide tooth comb is gentle on the hair and helps avoid breakage, especially on curly or textured hair.

2. Tail Comb (Rat-Tail Comb)

Purpose: Parting and sectioning hair.

Why It's Important: Clean, even sections are key to creating professional-looking braids. The pointed end of the tail comb helps in making precise parts, whether for intricate cornrows or simple three-strand braids.

3. Clips or Hair Sectioning Clamps

Purpose: Holding sections of hair in place while working on a braid.

Why It's Important: Keeping hair organized as you braid helps maintain focus on one section at a time, reducing the risk of tangling and uneven braiding.

4. Elastic Hair Ties (Small and Large)

Purpose: Securing the ends of braids or holding sections temporarily.

Why It's Important: Elastic ties help secure the braid once finished, ensuring it stays in place throughout the day. Small, snag-free elastics are best for securing the ends without damaging hair.

5. Hair Moisturizer or Leave-In Conditioner

Purpose: Keeping hair hydrated and smooth during braiding.

Why It's Important: Well-moisturized hair is less prone to breakage and frizzing, making it easier to braid. Applying a leave-in conditioner also helps the hair maintain its natural elasticity during the braiding process.

6. Edge Control Gel or Pomade

Purpose: Smoothing down flyaways and taming edges around the hairline.

Why It's Important: A clean finish is key to polished braids, and edge control gel helps manage any loose hairs for a sleeker look, especially for styles that involve intricate parts or cornrows.

7. Spray Bottle (Water)

Purpose: Re-moisturizing hair as needed during the braiding process.

Why It's Important: Braiding is easier on slightly damp hair, as it becomes more pliable and easier to manipulate. A spray bottle ensures hair doesn't dry out while working, particularly with longer styles.

8. Bristle Brush

Purpose: Smoothing hair into place before or during braiding.

Why It's Important: A bristle brush is excellent for gathering hair smoothly into tight braids and taming any stray hairs for a neater look. It can also help distribute product evenly through the hair.

9. Hair Bonnets or Silk Scarves (For Post-Braiding)

Purpose: Protecting braids while sleeping or during downtime.

Why It's Important: To maintain the longevity and neatness of your braids, covering them with a silk or satin bonnet or scarf prevents friction, which can cause frizzing or loosening of the braids overnight.

10. Scalp Oil or Serum

Purpose: Hydrating the scalp and promoting healthy hair growth during the life of the braid.

Why It's Important: Braiding can sometimes put strain on the scalp, so using oils like jojoba, tea tree, or coconut oil helps maintain scalp health and prevents dryness or irritation.

***Note:** Having the right tools is crucial for achieving clean, professional braids while protecting hair health. Whether you're braiding at home or in a professional setting, these tools will help ensure that the process is smooth, efficient, and enjoyable.*

Chapter 3

How to Prepare Hair for Braiding

Proper preparation of the hair before braiding is crucial for achieving neat, long-lasting braids while minimizing damage. Prepping the hair ensures it's manageable, well-hydrated, and free from tangles, making the braiding process easier and more comfortable. Here's a step-by-step guide on how to get your hair ready for braiding:

1. Cleanse the Hair

Step: Start with freshly washed hair.

Why It's Important: Clean hair prevents product buildup and oil from weighing down the braids. Braiding with dirty hair can lead to scalp irritation, increased frizz, and reduced braid longevity.

Tip: Use a sulfate-free shampoo for a gentle cleanse, particularly if you have textured or curly hair, to avoid stripping the hair of essential moisture.

2. Condition and Detangle

Step: Apply a deep conditioner or a rich, moisturizing conditioner to hydrate and soften the hair.

Why It's Important: Conditioning ensures the hair is moisturized and easier to work with, reducing the risk of breakage during the braiding process.

Detangle: After conditioning, use a wide-tooth comb or detangling brush to gently remove any knots or tangles. Start from the ends and work your way up to the roots.

Tip: Use a leave-in conditioner for extra hydration, especially if your hair is prone to dryness. This helps keep the hair soft and manageable throughout the braiding process.

3. Dry the Hair

Step: Depending on your hair type and the style of braid you want, you can either air dry or blow-dry your hair.

Why It's Important: Damp hair is more fragile, and braiding wet hair can lead to breakage, especially for those with fine or fragile hair. Drying the hair also helps lock in moisture and makes it easier to control during braiding.

For Straight/Loose Curls: Blow-dry the hair on a low to medium heat setting to smooth and stretch it out.

For Curly/Coily Hair: Consider blow-drying with a heat protectant to stretch the curls slightly. Alternatively, you can braid or twist the hair while it's damp and let it air dry for a more natural texture before re-braiding.

4. Moisturize the Hair

Step: Apply a leave-in conditioner or a light hair oil, such as argan or jojoba oil, to seal in moisture and protect the hair during the braiding process.

Why It's Important: Braiding can lead to dryness, particularly on the ends of the hair, so keeping the hair well-moisturized ensures it stays healthy throughout the lifespan of the braids.

Tip: Use the "LOC method" (Leave-in, Oil, Cream) for textured or coily hair types to layer and lock in maximum moisture.

5. Stretch the Hair (Optional)

Step: Depending on the braid style and hair texture, stretching the hair can help prevent tangles and create a smoother, longer-lasting braid.

Methods:

Blow-drying: Use a blow dryer on a low setting to stretch out curls or kinks.

Banding Method: Use small hair elastics to section off damp hair, wrapping elastics down the length of each section to gently stretch the hair as it dries.

Twisting/Braiding: You can also stretch hair by loosely braiding or twisting it and letting it dry overnight.

6. Section the Hair

Step: Use a tail comb to divide the hair into sections according to the desired braid style.

Why It's Important: Clean, precise parting is key to creating neat, professional-looking braids. Well-sectioned hair also ensures that braiding is organized and less stressful.

Tip: Clip or tie off sections you aren't working on to keep them out of the way.

7. Apply Edge Control (Optional)

Step: For a sleeker, more polished look, especially around the hairline, apply edge control gel or pomade.

Why It's Important: Taming flyaways and frizz around the edges of the hair helps create a cleaner, more defined braid pattern.

Tip: Use a small bristle brush or toothbrush to smooth the edges for better control and precision.

8. Prepare Hair Extensions (If Applicable)

Step: If you're using hair extensions, such as synthetic braiding hair, prepare it by detangling and sectioning it beforehand.

Why It's Important: Prepping the extensions ensures smooth and seamless integration with your natural hair, giving you more control during the braiding process.

Tip: *Match the texture and color of the extension hair with your natural hair for a more cohesive look.*

9. Check Hair and Scalp Condition

Step: Before starting, ensure that both your hair and scalp are healthy and free from irritation. If you experience any scalp issues (such as dandruff, dryness, or irritation), address them with a soothing scalp treatment before braiding.

Why It's Important: A healthy scalp is crucial for comfortable, long-lasting braids. Braiding on an unhealthy scalp can cause further irritation or discomfort.

Note: Preparing your hair properly for braiding ensures that it is healthy, moisturized, and free of tangles, making the braiding process easier and ensuring longer-lasting, neat results. By following these steps, you can reduce damage, promote hair health, and create braids that look polished and professional.

A. Understanding Hair Types and How They Affect Braiding Techniques

Hair type plays a significant role in how braids are created, maintained, and styled. Different hair types respond differently to tension, product use, and braiding techniques, so understanding your hair's texture and properties is crucial for achieving the best results. This guide explores various hair types and provides tips on how they affect braiding.

1. The Hair Typing System

Hair types are generally categorized based on the curl pattern and texture. The most common classification system breaks hair down into four categories:

- Type 1: Straight
- Type 2: Wavy
- Type 3: Curly
- Type 4: Coily/Kinky

Each type has its own set of challenges and advantages when it comes to braiding. Below is a breakdown of how different hair types affect braiding techniques and the considerations for each.

2. Type 1: Straight Hair

Characteristics:

- Straight, smooth texture with little to no curl pattern.

- Hair often has a natural sheen but may lack volume.

- Tends to get oily faster than curly or textured hair.

Impact on Braiding:

Advantages: Straight hair is generally easier to manipulate and section, which makes it ideal for clean, precise braiding.

Challenges: Because straight hair is smooth and slippery, braids may not hold as well without the use of grip-enhancing products or elastics. It can unravel easily if not secured properly.

Braiding Tips:

1. Use texture spray: Applying a texturizing spray or mousse adds grip and volume, making the hair easier to braid and helping the braids hold longer.

2. Tighter tension: Keep the braid tight to ensure it stays intact throughout the day.

3. Secure with elastics: Use small, clear hair elastics to secure the ends to prevent the braid from unraveling.

3. Type 2: Wavy Hair

Characteristics:

- Hair that has a loose wave or "S" pattern.
- Often a mix between straight and curly textures, with varying degrees of volume and frizz.

Impact on Braiding:

Advantages: The natural texture of wavy hair provides some grip, making it easier to braid compared to straight hair. Braids tend to look more voluminous and textured.

Challenges: Wavy hair can become frizzy, especially in humid conditions, and the waves may cause uneven tension during braiding.

Braiding Tips:

1. Detangle before braiding: Use a wide-tooth comb to gently detangle hair to prevent knots while braiding.
2. Moisturize to reduce frizz: Apply a lightweight leave-in conditioner or anti-frizz serum to tame frizz and smooth the hair's texture before braiding.
3. Loose, boho styles: Wavy hair works well with looser braids, like a messy fishtail or boho-style side braid, which embrace the hair's natural texture.

4. Type 3: Curly Hair

Characteristics:

- Well-defined curls, ranging from loose ringlets to tight spirals.
- Curly hair tends to be more voluminous but can also be prone to frizz and dryness.

Impact on Braiding:

Advantages: The natural curl pattern provides ample grip, which helps braids stay in place longer without needing as much product. Curly hair adds texture and volume to braids, giving them a fuller appearance.

Challenges: Curly hair can tangle easily, making it harder to section and braid neatly. It also tends to dry out quickly, which can lead to breakage if braided too tightly.

Braiding Tips:

1. Moisturize thoroughly: Apply a hydrating leave-in conditioner or curl cream before braiding to lock in moisture and reduce frizz.
2. Detangle with care: Gently detangle the hair with a wide-tooth comb or fingers, starting from the ends and working your way up to the roots.

3. Section carefully: Curly hair can create uneven sections if not parted correctly, so use a tail comb to create clean, defined sections before braiding.

4. Protective styles: Curly hair responds well to protective braiding styles like cornrows or box braids, which help reduce breakage and keep the hair tangle-free for longer periods.

5. Type 4: Coily/Kinky Hair

Characteristics:

- Tight, densely packed coils or kinks.
- Hair is often dry and more fragile, with a tendency to shrink significantly when not stretched.
- Has the most volume but can also be prone to breakage and tangling.

Impact on Braiding:

Advantages: Coily hair has a lot of texture and natural grip, making it ideal for intricate braiding patterns like cornrows, box braids, or twists. Braids tend to last longer and look more voluminous.

Challenges: The tight curl pattern makes it more prone to breakage, especially if the hair is dry or the braids are too tight. It also requires more maintenance to ensure the scalp remains moisturized.

Braiding Tips:

1. Deep condition regularly: Use a deep conditioning treatment before braiding to restore moisture and improve elasticity.
2. Stretch the hair: For easier braiding, stretch the hair using a blow-dryer or banding method to reduce shrinkage and make the hair more manageable.
3. Use scalp oil: Apply a light scalp oil during and after braiding to keep the scalp hydrated and reduce itching or irritation.

4. Protective styling: Coily hair is especially well-suited for protective styles like box braids, twists, or knotless braids, which help protect the hair from environmental damage and promote growth.

General Tips for All Hair Types

1. Avoid Tight Braids: Regardless of hair type, braiding too tightly can lead to tension, breakage, and even hair loss (traction alopecia). Always aim for a comfortable tension that keeps the braid secure without pulling on the scalp.

2. Choose the Right Products: Tailor your products to your hair type. Use anti-frizz serums for wavy or curly hair, and opt for lightweight oils for coily hair to keep it hydrated.

3. Moisturize and Protect: Regularly moisturize your hair to maintain its health,

and use satin or silk scarves to protect your braids at night.

Each hair type presents its own unique challenges and advantages when it comes to braiding. By understanding your specific hair texture and needs, you can choose the right braiding techniques and products to ensure your braids are not only beautiful but also healthy and long-lasting. Whether your hair is straight, wavy, curly, or coily, with the proper preparation and care, you can create stunning braids that highlight your hair's natural beauty.

B. Basics of Hair Sectioning, Grip, and Tension

Mastering the fundamentals of hair sectioning, grip, and tension is essential for achieving neat, professional looking braids. Whether you are working on simple three-strand braids or more complex styles, understanding how to properly section hair, maintain grip, and control tension will ensure that your braids are secure, uniform, and comfortable. Let's break down these three core elements:

A. Hair Sectioning

Sectioning hair properly is crucial for achieving organized and balanced braids. Clean, precise sections ensure that the braids are even and aesthetically pleasing.

1. Why Hair Sectioning Matters:

Symmetry: Proper sectioning ensures that each braid or row looks balanced and uniform.

Manageability: Working with smaller, well-defined sections makes braiding easier, especially with thicker or textured hair.

Neatness: Clean parting reduces the risk of stray hairs and gives the braid a polished, professional look.

2. How to Section Hair:

Tools: You'll need a rat-tail comb (tail comb) for precise parting and sectioning clips or hair ties to keep unused sections out of the way.

Step by Step Process:

i. **Start with detangled hair:** Make sure the hair is thoroughly detangled with a wide-tooth comb to avoid knots and tangles.

ii. **Identify your parting style:** Depending on the braid (e.g., cornrows, French braids, or box braids), decide on the parting style. You can do straight, diagonal, or zigzag partings depending on the look you want.

iii. **Part in manageable sections:** Use the pointed end of the tail comb to create clean partings. Part hair from the scalp to the ends, and secure the sections you are not working on with clips or ties.

iv. **Ensure even sections:** For braids that require equal parts (like box braids), make sure each section is evenly sized to avoid uneven or lopsided braids.

3. Pro Tips for Sectioning:

- **Work in rows:** For organized styles like cornrows or box braids, part the hair in horizontal or vertical rows first, then subdivide each row into smaller sections.
- **Keep sections tight:** Ensure that the section of hair you're working with is smooth and pulled taut before braiding to avoid bumps or loose strands.
- **Check mirrors:** If braiding your own hair, use multiple mirrors or ask someone to check the back to ensure even parting.

B. Grip

Grip refers to how you hold and control the hair while braiding. A good grip ensures that each braid is tight and secure, leading to a neater, longer-lasting style.

1. Why Grip is Important:

- Prevents braids from loosening: Proper grip ensures that the braid doesn't unravel or loosen throughout the day.
- Creates clean, defined braids: A firm grip helps maintain uniformity throughout the braid, making it look sleek and professional.
- Maintains control: Good grip helps you maintain control over each strand, preventing flyaways or tangling as you braid.

2. How to Achieve the Right Grip:

- Start with small sections: Use manageable sections of hair that are appropriate for the braid size you are attempting. Trying to work with too much hair at once can make it difficult to maintain control.
- Hold strands between your fingers: As you braid, hold the strands firmly between your thumb and index or middle finger. The hand

holding the braid should keep the strands
taut, while the other hand works to cross the
sections over.

- Adjust your grip: Keep adjusting your grip
  as you move down the length of the braid,
  maintaining even tension. As the braid gets
  longer, shift your fingers closer to the braid
  to maintain control.

3. Pro Tips for Improving Grip:

- Dry hands: If your hands are too slippery,
  use a small amount of cornstarch or grip-
  enhancing spray to improve your hold on the
  hair.
- Use hair products: On straight or fine hair,
  applying texture spray or a light mousse can
  help increase grip by adding some texture
  and preventing the hair from slipping out of
  your fingers.
- Practice with smaller braids: Start practicing
  on smaller braids to get used to maintaining

a tight grip, then work up to more complex styles.

C. Tension

Tension refers to how tightly or loosely you pull the hair while braiding. Correct tension is critical for achieving braids that are secure without causing discomfort or damage to the hair and scalp.

1. Why Tension is Important:

- Prevents scalp damage: Too much tension can cause discomfort, scalp irritation, or even hair loss due to traction alopecia. Proper tension protects both the hair and the scalp.
- Ensures braid longevity: Consistent tension throughout the braid helps it last longer, as loose braids tend to unravel or frizz more quickly.

- Creates uniform braids: Consistent tension keeps the braid tight and neat from root to end, resulting in a more polished look.

2. How to Control Tension:

- Balanced pull: As you braid, apply an even amount of tension to each strand. Avoid pulling too hard at the roots, but ensure that the braid is snug enough to stay in place.
- Check the scalp: While braiding, check in with the person (or yourself) to ensure there is no discomfort or tightness at the scalp. If the braid feels too tight, loosen your grip slightly and continue braiding with lighter tension.
- Even throughout: Make sure the tension is consistent from the roots to the ends. Inconsistencies in tension can cause the braid to look bulky at one point and too loose at another.

3. Pro Tips for Managing Tension:

- Use scalp oil: For protective styles like cornrows or box braids, applying a light scalp oil (such as jojoba or tea tree) can soothe the scalp and make it easier to manage tension without discomfort.

- Looser for sensitive scalps: If braiding for someone with a sensitive scalp, use looser tension to avoid pain or irritation, but make sure the braid is still secure.

- Don't pull too tightly: While tighter braids last longer, too much tension can weaken the hair follicles, especially around the hairline. Maintain a balance between tightness and comfort.

Note: Become skilled at the basics of hair sectioning, grip, and tension is key to creating neat, long-lasting braids while protecting the hair and scalp. Proper sectioning allows for clean, organized braiding, a good grip ensures control and neatness, and managing tension keeps braids secure without causing discomfort. These foundational skills, combined with practice, will help you braid with precision and confidence.

Chapter 4

Foundational Techniques for Hair Braiding

Mastering the foundational techniques of hair braiding is the first step toward creating more complex and creative braid styles. In this section, we'll cover the basics of essential braiding methods that serve as building blocks for more advanced techniques.

A. The Three-Strand Braids and Their Variations

The three-strand braid is the most basic and widely known braiding technique. It serves as the foundation for more complex braiding styles. Once you've mastered the classic three-strand braid, you can explore several variations, such as the side braid and double braids, to diversify your styling options. These styles are versatile, suitable for everyday wear or special occasions, and work well with various hair types.

1. Classic Three-Strand Braid

The classic three-strand braid is a simple yet elegant braid that involves alternating three sections of hair by crossing them over one another. It's ideal for a neat, polished look and can be done on any hair length, from shoulder length to long hair.

Here is the image of a classic three-strand braid.

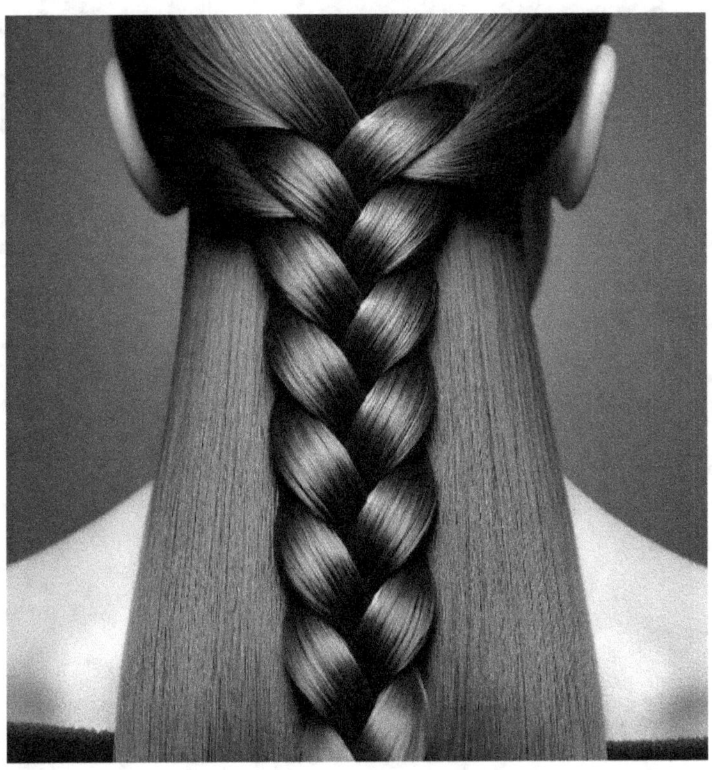

Instructions:

Step 1. Brush and detangle:

Start by brushing the hair to remove any tangles or knots. This ensures smooth and even braids.

Step 2. Divide the hair into three sections:

Gather all the hair and divide it into three equal parts: left, middle, and right.

Step 3. Cross the right section over the middle:

Take the right section of hair and cross it over the middle section. The right section is now the new middle.

Step 4. Cross the left section over the middle:

Take the left section of hair and cross it over the new middle section.

Step 5. Repeat the process:

Continue crossing the right and left sections over the middle, alternating each time, until you reach the end of the hair.

Step 6. Secure the braid:

Once you've braided all the way down, secure the end with a small elastic band to keep it in place.

Tips for the Classic Braid:

1. Tension: Keep a consistent tension throughout the braid to avoid it being too loose or uneven.
2. Practice symmetry: Ensure the sections are even from the start to achieve a uniform braid.
3. Finish with style: You can leave the braid as-is for a classic look, or pull gently on the braid's edges to make it appear fuller and more voluminous.

2. Side Braid

The side braid is a stylish variation of the classic three-strand braid that begins on one side of the head and rests over the shoulder. It's perfect for creating a relaxed, casual look while still keeping the hair neat and contained.

Here is the image of a classic three-strand side braid.

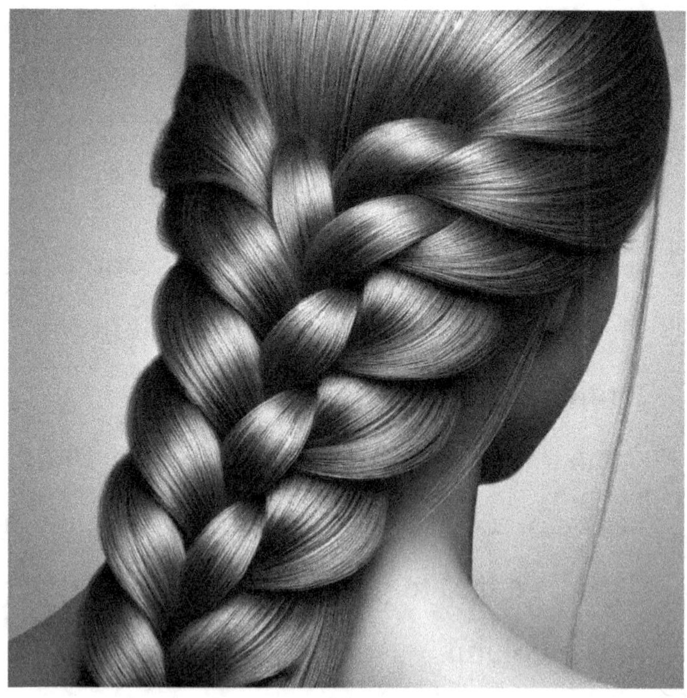

Instructions:

Step 1. Part the hair:

Part your hair to one side, gathering all of it over one shoulder.

Step 2. Divide the hair into three sections:

Just like the classic braid, divide the hair into three equal parts.

Step 3. Begin braiding:

Start by crossing the right section over the middle, followed by the left section over the middle.

Step 4. Braid down the length:

Continue the process until you reach the ends of your hair. Because the braid is positioned over the shoulder, it can be done slightly looser for a more relaxed look.

Step 5. Secure the braid:

Tie the end of the braid with an elastic band to keep it in place.

Tips for the Side Braid:

1. Loose or tight: A looser side braid creates a more bohemian, laid-back vibe, while a tighter braid looks sleek and polished.
2. Add texture: For a more textured look, gently pull on the braid's edges to loosen it and create a messier appearance.
3. Face framing: Leave out a few face-framing strands for a soft, romantic look.

3. Double Braids (Pigtail Braids)

Double braids, also known as pigtail braids, are two three-strand braids created on either side of the head. This style is fun, youthful, and ideal for an active day or casual outing. It's also a great protective style for natural hair, keeping it neatly tucked away.

Here is the image of double braids (pigtail braids).

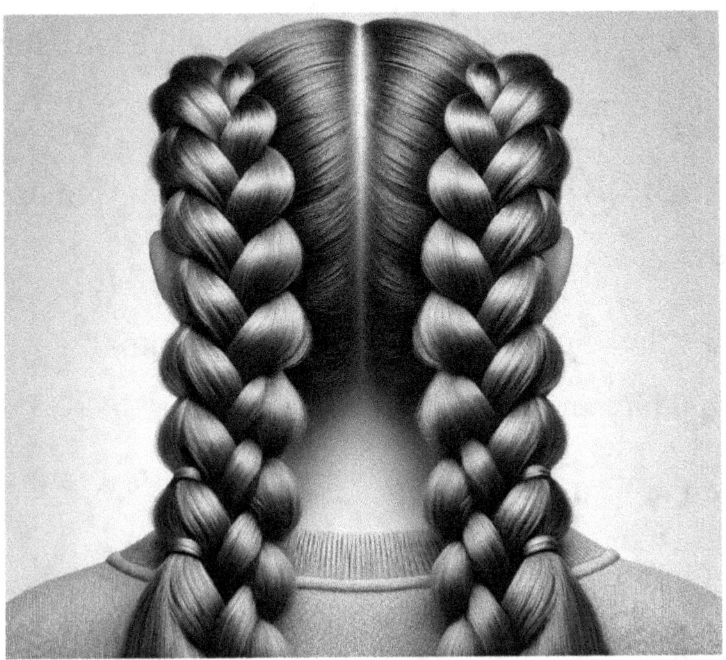

Instructions:

Step 1. Part the hair down the middle:

Use a tail comb to create a clean center part,
dividing the hair into two equal sections (left and
right).

Step 2. Clip one side:

To keep one section out of the way while working on the other, clip or tie one side.

Step 3. Divide the hair into three sections on one side:

Take the unpinned section and split it into three equal parts near the nape of the neck.

Step 4. Start braiding:

Begin braiding by crossing the right section over the middle, followed by the left section over the middle. Repeat this process, working down to the ends of the hair.

Step 5. Secure the first braid:

Once the braid is complete, tie it with an elastic.

Step 6. Repeat on the other side:

Unclip the other section of hair and repeat the same braiding process.

Step 7. Final touches:

Once both braids are complete, you can leave them tight for a sleek look or loosen them for a more relaxed style.

Tips for Double Braids:

1. Even parting: Ensure the center part is clean and even to maintain balance and symmetry in the braids.
2. Play with positioning: You can place the braids lower at the nape for a more casual look or start higher for a more structured style.
3. Accessorize: Add ribbons, beads, or colored elastics to give the style a playful or customized touch.

Variations and Styling Ideas

Messy Braids: For a more casual and undone look, gently pull on the sections of the braid to create a messier, fuller appearance. This works especially well for side braids and double braids.

Accessorized Braids: Enhance your braids with accessories like ribbons, flowers, or small hair clips. You can weave a ribbon through the braid for a pop of color or add small decorative clips for a festive touch.

Braid into a Bun: For a more polished style, braid the hair and then twist it into a bun at the nape of the neck, securing it with bobby pins.

Note: The classic three-strand braid is the cornerstone of braiding, providing a solid foundation for more intricate styles. Its variations, such as the side braid and double braids, offer versatility and can be adapted for various occasions and preferences. Once you've mastered these styles, you'll have the skills to create a wide range of braided looks, from casual and relaxed to sleek and formal.

Troubleshooting Common Beginner Issues in Braiding

When learning to braid, beginners often encounter challenges that can lead to uneven braids, loose strands, or braids that don't hold up well. These issues are normal and easily fixable with practice and attention to technique. Here's a guide to help you troubleshoot some of the most common problems and ensure that your braids turn out neat and secure.

1. Uneven Braids

Problem: Your braid looks uneven, with some sections appearing thicker or thinner than others, making the braid look lopsided or messy.

Causes:

- Uneven sectioning: The three sections of hair may not be divided equally at the start, causing one strand to dominate the others.

- Inconsistent tension: If one hand pulls more tightly than the other, the braid can become uneven.

Solution:

- Start with equal sections: Before you begin braiding, carefully divide the hair into three equal parts. Using a tail comb can help you make cleaner, more even sections.
- Check your tension: Make sure you are pulling the strands with consistent tension throughout the braid. Both hands should apply the same amount of pressure to keep the braid balanced. A good way to test this is to gently tug on the braid after a few passes to ensure it's even.
- Practice symmetrical braiding: Try braiding slowly at first to focus on even hand movements. With practice, your hands will get used to moving in sync.

2. Loose Strands

Problem: Hair strands slip out of the braid, making it look messy or unkempt.

Causes:

- Not gripping the hair tightly enough: Loose grip on the strands allows them to slip out of place.
- Hair too smooth or slippery: Hair that is very straight or fine tends to slip more easily, especially if it's freshly washed or not texturized.

Solution:

- Increase grip: Make sure you're holding the strands firmly as you cross them over each other. Keep the braid tight but not so tight that it becomes uncomfortable.
- Use texturizing products: If your hair is naturally slippery or fine, apply a texturizing spray, mousse, or a light dry shampoo

before braiding. These products give the hair more texture, making it easier to grip and hold in place.

- Smooth as you go: Before crossing each strand over, run your fingers along the section to smooth it out and reduce frizz. This keeps the braid cleaner and more contained.

3. Braids Coming Loose or Unraveling

Problem: Your braid becomes loose and starts to unravel shortly after finishing it, especially at the end or along the length of the braid.

Causes:

- Insufficient tension: The braid may be too loose, allowing it to fall apart more easily.
- Weak or missing hair ties: Not securing the end of the braid tightly enough can cause it to unravel.

Solution:

- Tighten the braid: Keep tension consistent throughout the braiding process, making sure each crossover is firm and snug.

- Secure with a strong hair tie: Use a small, strong elastic to tie the end of the braid tightly. Avoid using hair ties that slip off easily, and make sure the braid is secured firmly to prevent unraveling.

- Finish with hairspray: For extra hold, use a light mist of hairspray to set the braid in place, especially if you're wearing it throughout the day or for an event.

4. Frizz or Flyaways

Problem: Small hairs stick out of the braid, giving it a frizzy or unpolished look.

Causes:

- Hair not smoothed before braiding: Frizz can occur when hair isn't smoothed down before braiding.

- Damaged or broken hair: Damaged hair can create flyaways due to split ends or broken strands.

Solution:

- Use smoothing products: Apply a small amount of leave-in conditioner, serum, or lightweight oil to the hair before braiding. This helps smooth out frizz and adds shine to the braid.
- Brush or comb the hair first: Make sure the hair is thoroughly brushed or combed before starting the braid. For curly or textured hair, using a detangling spray or leave-in conditioner can help reduce frizz.
- Tame flyaways with gel: For a sleeker look, use a small amount of edge control gel or styling cream to smooth down flyaways. Use a fine-tooth comb or a toothbrush to carefully brush the hairs into place.

5. Braid Too Tight

Problem: The braid is too tight, causing discomfort or tension on the scalp.

Causes:

- Over-tightening the braid: Pulling too hard while braiding can put excessive tension on the scalp and hair.
- Improper grip: Holding the hair too firmly while braiding can lead to tightness.

Solution:

- Relax your grip: Hold the strands firmly but not too tightly. You should feel the braid is secure without pulling on the scalp.
- Check for tension as you go: As you braid, check the tightness by gently touching the braid and scalp. If it feels too tight, loosen your grip slightly.
- Leave some slack at the scalp: When starting a braid at the scalp (like in French or

Dutch braids), make sure to leave a small amount of slack to avoid putting too much pressure on the hairline or scalp.

6. Braid Not Lasting Throughout the Day

Problem: Your braid falls apart or becomes frizzy and loose over the course of the day.

Causes:

- Improper tension or grip: Loose braiding techniques can cause the braid to lose its structure.
- Environmental factors: Humidity, wind, or physical activity can cause a braid to unravel or frizz.

Solution:

- Set the braid with product: Use hairspray or a setting spray after finishing the braid to help it hold its shape throughout the day. Opt for an anti-humidity spray if you live in a humid climate.

- Braid tighter if needed: A slightly tighter braid at the start will loosen naturally over the day but will still hold its shape. Don't make it so tight that it causes discomfort, but secure enough to last.

- Use smaller sections for better hold: For longer-lasting braids, use smaller, more precise sections of hair. This helps the braid maintain its shape for longer.

Most common braiding issues, like uneven braids or loose strands, can be fixed with better sectioning, more consistent tension, and the right products. With practice and attention to these small details, your braiding skills will improve, and your braids will stay secure, neat, and polished. Don't be discouraged by early mistakes—every braid is a step toward mastery!

Chapter 5

Advanced Braiding Techniques

Once you've mastered the basics of braiding, you're ready to take on more advanced styles like French, Dutch, and Fishtail braids. These techniques build on the foundational three-strand braid but involve incorporating additional sections of hair and using different crossing patterns to create more intricate, visually stunning designs.

A. Understanding the Structure and Mechanics of the French, Dutch, and Fishtail Braids

Each of these advanced braiding techniques has a distinct structure and mechanics. Here's a breakdown of how they work:

1. French Braid

Structure: The French braid starts at the crown of the head and lies flat against the scalp. As you braid, you incorporate hair from the sides of the head into the braid, resulting in a smooth, cohesive style that pulls all the hair neatly back.

Mechanics:

- Three-Strand Base: Like the classic three-strand braid, the French braid begins with three sections of hair.
- Adding Hair: The key difference is that, as you cross the sections, you continuously add small sections of hair from the sides of your head to the outer sections before crossing them over the middle.
- Building from the Top Down: You start near the hairline and work your way down the scalp, gradually incorporating all of the hair.

Here is the image of a classic French braid.

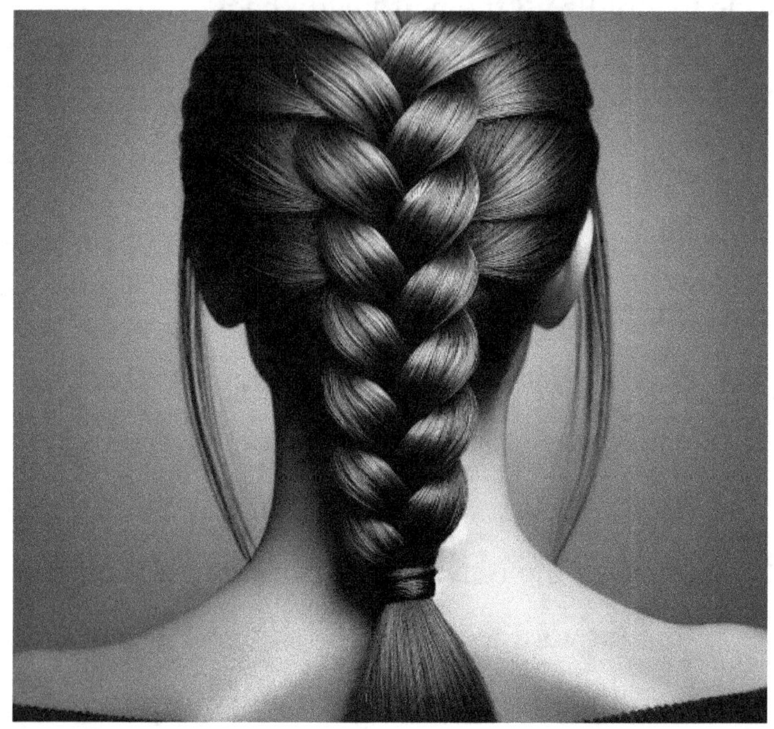

How It Works:

Step 1. Start with a Section at the Crown:
Separate a section of hair at the crown into three
equal strands.

Step 2. Begin a Regular Braid: Cross the right
section over the middle, then the left over the
middle, as in a standard three-strand braid.

Step 3. Add Hair as You Go: As you continue, gather a small piece of hair from the right side of your head and add it to the right strand before crossing it over the middle. Repeat with the left side.

Step 4. Continue to the Nape: Keep adding hair to each section until you reach the nape of the neck. Once all the hair is gathered, finish with a regular three-strand braid down the length of the hair.

Step 5. Secure with an Elastic: Tie the braid with a small elastic to keep it intact.

Key Mechanics:

Tension Control: To keep the braid looking polished and secure, maintain consistent tension throughout, pulling the hair snugly as you add new sections.

Symmetry: Be sure to add equal amounts of hair to each side to keep the braid balanced and symmetrical.

2. Dutch Braid

Structure: The Dutch braid, often referred to as an "inside-out" or "reverse French braid," stands out from the head rather than lying flat. The mechanics are similar to the French braid, but the strands are crossed under the middle section, which creates a raised, 3D effect.

Mechanics:

Reverse Three-Strand: Like the French braid, the Dutch braid uses three sections, but instead of crossing the outer sections over the middle, you cross them under the middle.

Incorporating Hair: Just like the French braid, you add sections of hair from the sides as you work your way down.

Here is the image of a classic Dutch braid.

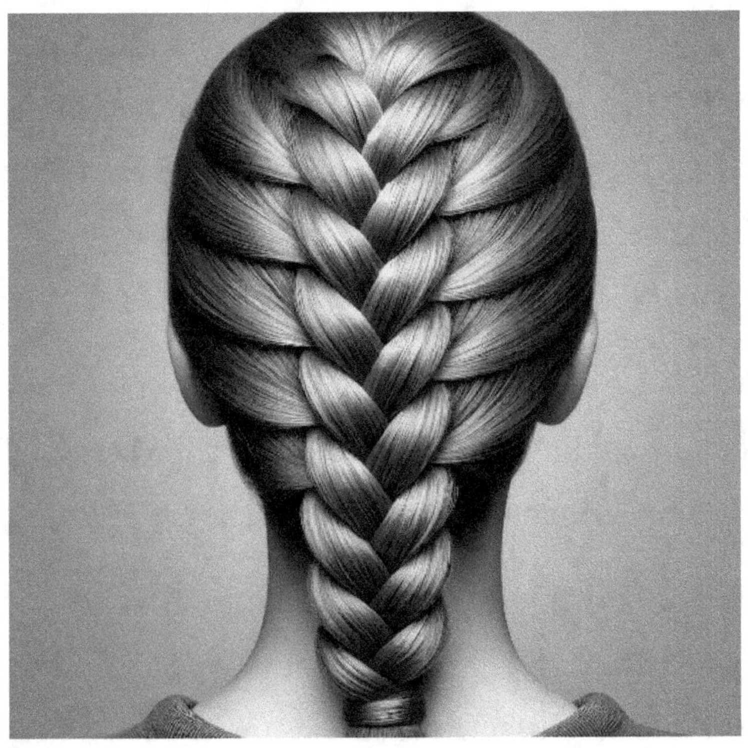

How It Works:

Step 1. Start with a Section at the Crown:
Separate a section of hair at the crown into three equal parts.

Step 2. Cross Under the Middle: Take the right section and cross it under the middle section, then take the left section and cross it under the new middle.

Step 3. Add Hair to the Sections: Before each new cross, gather a small section of hair from the right side and add it to the right strand, then cross it under the middle. Repeat on the left side.

Step 4. Continue Down the Scalp: As you continue adding hair from both sides, the braid will take on its signature raised appearance.

Step 5. Finish with a Regular Three-Strand Braid: Once all the hair is incorporated, complete the braid by crossing the strands under each other, and secure with an elastic.

Key Mechanics:

Underhand Motion: The main difference from the French braid is the underhand crossing motion, which creates the raised braid. Practice this motion to get used to the feel.

Tightness: The Dutch braid looks best when pulled tightly against the scalp to enhance the 3D effect.

3. Fishtail Braid

Structure: The fishtail braid has a more delicate, woven appearance and is created with only two sections of hair instead of three. The braid is made by taking small sections from each side and crossing them over, creating a pattern that resembles the scales of a fish.

Mechanics:

Two-Strand Weave: Unlike the three-strand technique used in French and Dutch braids, the fishtail braid divides the hair into two sections. Small pieces from each section are crossed over the middle, alternating sides to build the braid.

Gradual Tapering: The braid tapers down as it gets longer, creating a sleek, smooth look.

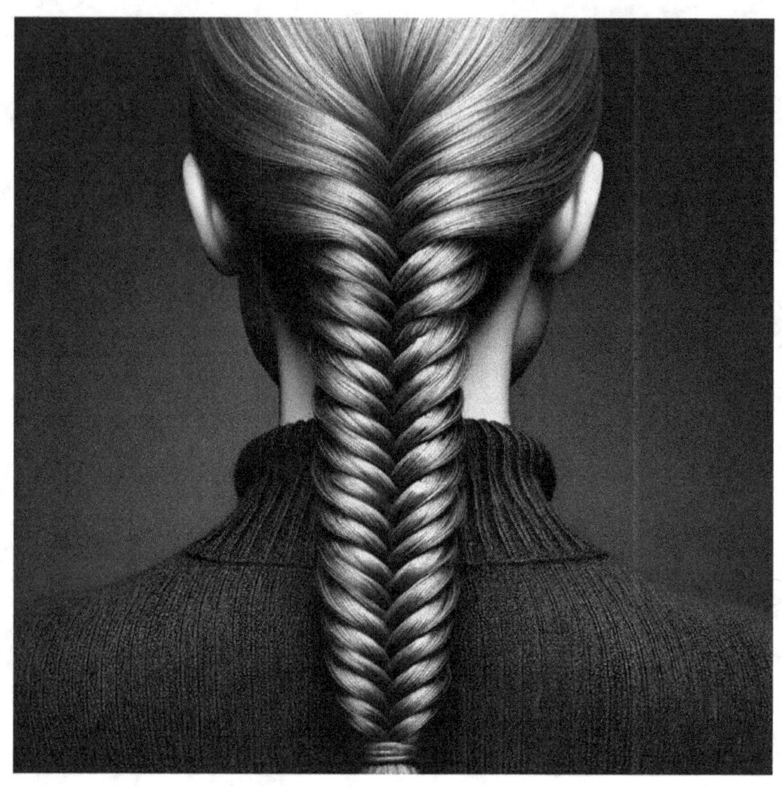

How It Works:

Step 1. Divide Hair into Two Sections: Separate the hair into two equal parts.

Step 2. Take a Small Strand from the Right: Grab a small piece of hair from the outer edge of the right section, and cross it over to join the left section.

Step 3. Take a Small Strand from the Left: Now take a small piece of hair from the outer edge of the left section, and cross it over to join the right section.

Step 4. Repeat the Process: Continue alternating, crossing small sections from one side to the other until you reach the end of the hair.

Step 5. Secure with an Elastic: Once the braid is complete, tie it off with a small elastic.

Key Mechanics:

Small Sections for Intricacy: The smaller the sections of hair you take from each side, the more detailed and intricate the braid will appear.

Loose or Tight: Fishtail braids can be worn tight for a sleek, polished look or loosened for a more bohemian, relaxed style by gently tugging on the sides of the braid.

The structure and mechanics of French, Dutch, and Fishtail braids all involve different crossing methods and techniques, resulting in distinct looks. The French braid is smooth and flat, while the Dutch braid adds a raised, textured appearance. The Fishtail braid, with its two-strand weave, offers a delicate, intricate look. Mastering these braids will open the door to endless creative styling possibilities!

B. Layered Instructions for Mastering Tightness and Symmetry in Braids

Tightness and symmetry are key to achieving clean, professional looking braids. Whether you're working on a three-strand braid, French braid, Dutch braid, or fishtail braid, mastering these elements will help your braids stay secure, look polished, and last longer. Here's a step by step guide that builds on basic techniques to help you control tension and create symmetrical braids.

Step 1: Preparing the Hair for Braiding

Achieving tightness and symmetry starts with how you prepare your hair.

Instructions:

1. Detangle the Hair Completely:

Use a wide-tooth comb to remove any knots or tangles. This helps create smooth, even sections that braid more easily and neatly.

2. Use the Right Products:

- For fine or slippery hair, apply a texturizing spray or mousse to add grip.
- For curly or coily hair, use a leave-in conditioner or a light oil to add moisture and smoothness, making it easier to control.

3. Section the Hair Properly:

Divide the hair into even sections using a tail comb. Clean parting lines ensure that your braid will be symmetrical and uniform.

Step 2: Achieving the Right Tightness

Instructions:

1. Start with Firm Control:

As you begin the braid, make sure your hands have a firm grip on the sections of hair. Hold the hair snugly between your thumb and index fingers.

2. Tighten at the Roots:

When starting a braid, especially with French or Dutch braids, make sure to braid close to the scalp. Keep the sections tight as you cross them over or under each other. This will help the braid stay secure and neat from the roots.

Tip: Don't pull too hard, especially around the edges or hairline, as this can cause discomfort or damage the hair (traction alopecia).

3. Maintain Consistent Tension:

As you braid down the length of the hair, continue to apply even tension to each section. The braid should feel tight enough to hold its shape but not so tight that it's painful or uncomfortable.

Check for Consistency: Periodically run your fingers over the braid to ensure the tightness is even from the top to the bottom. If one section feels looser, gently pull on the strand to tighten it.

4. Adjust as You Go:

If you notice that a section is looser than the others while braiding, pause and tighten it slightly before continuing. It's easier to fix tension issues as you braid rather than after you've finished.

Step 3: Ensuring Symmetry

Symmetry ensures your braid looks balanced and evenly proportioned on both sides. Uneven braids can look sloppy, but by focusing on balance throughout, you can ensure a clean, polished result.

Instructions:

1. Divide Sections Evenly:

When you divide the hair into sections, make sure each section is the same size. Uneven sections can cause the braid to look lopsided or bulky on one side.

Tip: Use your fingers or a comb to adjust and measure the thickness of each section as you divide it. Take your time during this step to avoid imbalance later.

2. Cross Sections Over/Under Evenly:

As you braid, focus on crossing each section in the same way every time. In a French braid, make sure the amount of hair added from each side is consistent, and in a Dutch braid, cross each section under the same way.

Maintain Consistent Distance: The sections should cross over or under each other at the same distance each time, so the braid pattern looks even.

3. Check for Alignment:

As you braid, take breaks to look in the mirror and check the alignment of the braid. This is especially important for French and Dutch braids, where symmetry is key to a sleek appearance.

Tip: If braiding your own hair, use a double mirror setup or ask for help to ensure symmetry from the back.

4. Mirror Each Side in Double Braids:

When creating double braids (like pigtails), start by parting the hair down the center. Make sure each section on both sides is identical. As you braid, ensure that the number of crossovers and tension are the same on both sides for a balanced look.

Step 4: Finishing the Braid with Tightness and Symmetry in Mind

The way you finish your braid plays a big role in how tight and symmetrical it looks overall.

Instructions:

1. Tighten as You Reach the Ends:

As you reach the end of the braid, you may notice that the sections become thinner and more difficult to control. Maintain the tension by pulling the sections tightly as you continue to cross them.

Tip: Use smaller hair ties to secure the braid more effectively without slipping.

2. Secure the End Firmly:

Tie the end of the braid with a strong, small elastic to ensure it doesn't unravel. You can also use a bit of hairspray on the ends for extra hold.

3. Adjust for Symmetry:

After finishing the braid, check the symmetry one last time. For French and Dutch braids, make sure the braid follows a straight path down the center of the scalp. For side braids or fishtail braids, ensure the braid sits evenly across your shoulder.

4. Gently Pancake the Braid (Optional):

If you want a fuller, softer look, gently pull on the edges of the braid (called "pancaking") to make it appear looser without affecting its overall tightness. This works particularly well for fishtail and Dutch braids.

Step 5: Practice Techniques for Mastering Tightness and Symmetry

Practice Drill 1: Tightness Control

Braid a small section of hair, paying attention to consistent tightness. Then undo it and re-braid with slightly more tension. Practice until you can achieve the same tightness throughout the braid without pulling too hard.

Practice Drill 2: Symmetry Check

Part your hair down the middle and practice creating two identical braids (pigtail braids). Take your time to ensure both sides are even and use a mirror to check your work. Keep practicing until both braids look symmetrical and balanced.

Troubleshooting Common Issues:

1. Loose Roots: If your braids are loose at the roots, try gripping the hair closer to the scalp as you begin the braid, and ensure you're pulling each section snugly from the start.

2. Uneven Strands: If you end up with uneven braid sections, take extra care when dividing the hair at the beginning. Using a comb can help you achieve cleaner, more symmetrical sections.

3. Braids Unraveling: If your braids unravel easily, secure them with tighter elastics and consider applying a light hairspray to hold them in place.

Mastering tightness and symmetry in braiding takes practice, patience, and a focus on detail. By controlling tension and ensuring even sectioning, you can create beautiful, balanced braids that are both comfortable and long-lasting. With consistent effort, these techniques will become second nature, and your braids will look professional and polished.

Chapter 6

Creative Braiding Styles

For those looking to take their braiding skills to the next level, creative braiding styles like crowns, halo braids, and waterfall braids offer sophisticated and beautiful options. These styles are perfect for special occasions, or when you want to add a unique flair to your everyday look. Here's an exploration of these creative braiding styles, with step by step instructions for mastering them.

A. Crown Braids: The Regal Style for Any Occasion

A crown braid is one of the most elegant and versatile braiding styles, perfect for both casual and formal occasions. This circular braid wraps around the head, giving a timeless, regal look. It can be created using a variety of braiding techniques, such as the Dutch braid or French braid, and offers endless opportunities for customization with accessories, textures, and volume.

1. Classic Dutch Crown Braid

The Dutch crown braid uses the Dutch braiding technique, which involves crossing the outer sections of the braid under the middle section. This creates a braid that stands out from the head, giving a raised, 3D effect. The braid is wrapped around the head, creating a "crown" that is both functional and stylish.

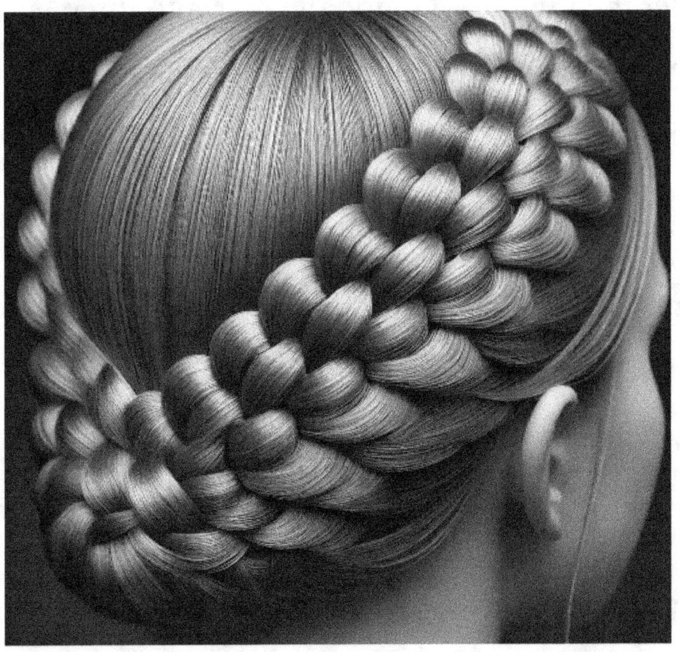

Above is the image of a classic Dutch crown braid.

Instructions:

Step 1. Part the Hair:

Start with a deep side part. This part will determine where your braid begins and ensures a natural flow around the head.

Step 2. Start Braiding Near the Nape:

Begin near the nape of the neck, on one side of the head, with a Dutch braid (crossing the strands under the middle). Divide the hair into three sections and start the braid, picking up hair from both sides as you move around the head.

Step 3. Work Your Way Around the Head:

Continue braiding along the perimeter of your hairline. Keep adding sections of hair to the braid as you move toward the top of the head and around the back. The Dutch braiding technique will create a raised braid that sits prominently on the scalp.

Step 4. Finish at the Starting Point:

When you complete the circle and reach the point where you began, finish with a simple three-strand braid down the remaining length of hair.

Step 5. Tuck and Pin:

Tuck the loose end of the braid under the starting point and secure it with bobby pins. Make sure the ends are hidden to maintain the seamless crown look.

Step 6. Loosen the Braid for Volume:

Gently pull on the edges of the braid to "pancake" it, making it appear fuller and softer. This step also gives the braid a more relaxed, bohemian feel.

Styling Tips:

- Textured or Smooth: You can create a sleek, polished version of the crown braid by smoothing the hair before braiding, or opt for a more textured, casual look by leaving

the hair slightly messy or using texturizing
spray.

- Accessory Ideas: Enhance the crown braid
with small flowers, jeweled pins, or ribbons
woven into the braid for special occasions
like weddings or festivals.

2. French Crown Braid

The French crown braid is similar to the Dutch
version but uses the French braiding technique,
where the outer sections are crossed over the
middle. This braid lies flatter against the head and
offers a subtler, sophisticated look.

Here is the image of the French crown braid.

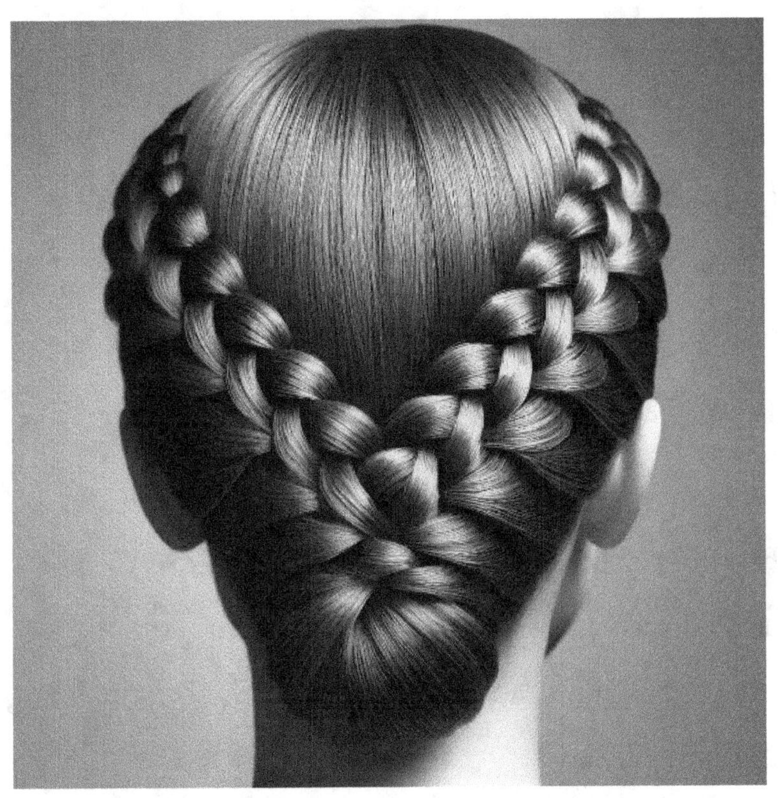

Instructions:

Step 1. Part and Section the Hair:

Start by parting the hair on one side. You can also part it down the middle if you prefer a symmetrical look. Divide the hair into three sections near the nape of the neck.

Step 2. Begin with a French Braid:

Starting near the ear or at the nape, begin a French braid, crossing the strands over the middle. As you braid, pull in sections from the sides to add volume and continue the braid around the head.

Step 3. Move Around the Crown:

As you braid, work your way up around the hairline, making sure to add even sections of hair as you go. Keep braiding until you've wrapped all the way around the head, ensuring the braid is snug but not too tight.

Step 4. Complete the Braid:

Once you have braided around the head and reach your starting point, finish with a regular three-strand braid. Tuck the end of the braid under the beginning and secure it with bobby pins.

Step 5. Refine the Look:

If you prefer a voluminous look, gently pull on the edges of the braid to loosen it. You can also use a light mist of hairspray to tame any flyaways.

Styling Tips:

- For a Sleek Finish: Keep the French crown braid tighter for a polished and formal style.
- Bohemian Vibe: For a softer, boho-inspired style, leave a few face-framing pieces loose and pull the braid to give it more volume and texture.

3. Double Crown Braid

The double crown braid consists of two braids wrapped around the head, creating an intricate layered effect. This style adds extra volume and detail, making it perfect for formal events.

Here is the image of the double crown braid.

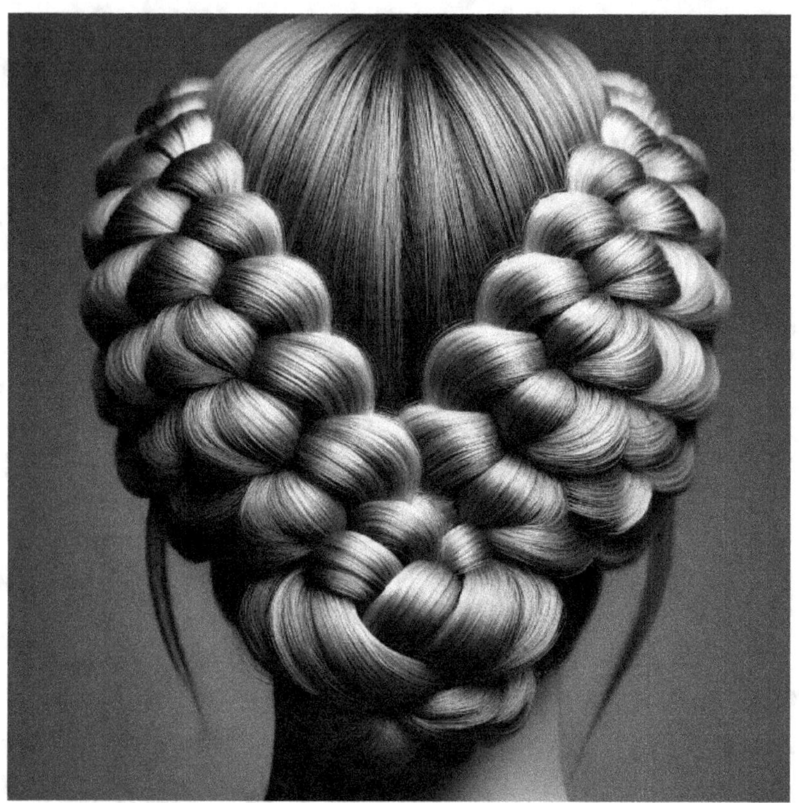

Instructions:

Step 1. Create a Part:

Part the hair down the middle, dividing it into two sections.

Step 2. Start Two Dutch or French Braids:

Start at the nape of the neck on one side and braid up toward the crown, using either a Dutch braid or a French braid. Repeat the same process on the other side.

Step 3. Wrap the First Braid Around the Head:

Once you finish the first braid, wrap it around the top of your head and secure it with bobby pins.

Step 4. Wrap the Second Braid:

Do the same with the second braid, crossing it over or under the first braid, depending on the desired effect.

Step 5. Tuck and Pin:

Tuck the ends of both braids neatly under each other and secure them with bobby pins.

Styling Tips:

- Maximize Volume: Pancake the braids by gently pulling on the edges to create a fuller look.

- Twist Variation: For a twist on this look, you can create one braid with a fishtail technique and the other with a Dutch braid for contrasting textures.

4. Crown Braid with Loose Waves

For a softer, more romantic look, a crown braid combined with loose waves is a stunning style. The braid frames the face while the loose waves add volume and flow.

Here is the image of a crown braid with loose waves.

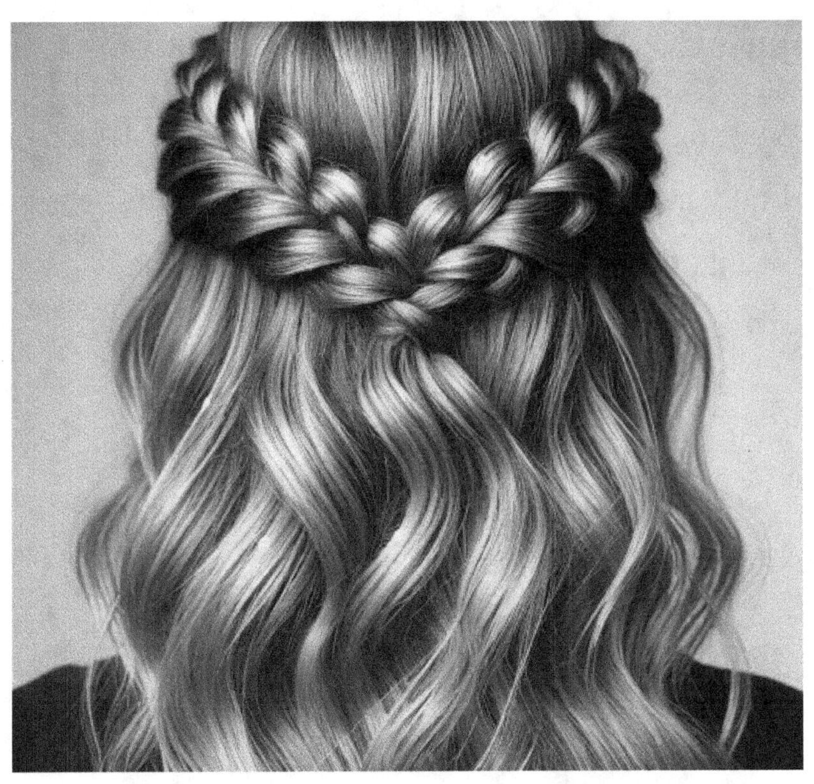

Instructions:

Step 1. Curl or Wave the Hair:

Before braiding, use a curling iron or wand to create soft waves throughout the hair. This gives the style more texture and movement.

Step 2. Create a French or Dutch Braid:

Starting at the ear, create a loose French or Dutch braid around the head. Make sure to keep it loose so that the braid blends in naturally with the waves.

Step 3. Secure and Style the Braid:

Once you finish the braid, tuck the end under the starting point and secure it with bobby pins.

Step 4. Blend the Braid with the Waves:

Gently pull on the braid to soften its appearance and blend it with the waves for a seamless, flowing look.

Styling Tips:

- Beachy Look: For a beachy, relaxed style, leave the braid slightly messy and the waves tousled.

- Sleek Waves: For a more formal look, keep the waves smooth and polished with a shine serum or hairspray.

Crown braids offer a range of styling options, from intricate and formal to relaxed and bohemian. They're versatile enough to suit various occasions, from weddings to music festivals. With the ability to customize the braid's texture, volume, and added accessories, crown braids can be adapted to reflect personal style while still maintaining a timeless, elegant look.

B. Halo Braids: The Angelic, Effortless Style

The halo braid is a stunning, circular braid that wraps around the head, similar to a crown braid, but typically sits higher on the head, creating a soft, angelic look. This braid is perfect for formal occasions, romantic settings, or when you want an ethereal, effortless appearance. The halo braid can be created using French or Dutch braiding techniques and can be styled in a variety of ways to suit different hair types and textures.

1. Classic Halo Braid

The classic halo braid encircles the head with a braid that is slightly looser and softer than the crown braid. It's a versatile style that can be dressed up or down and is perfect for medium to long hair.

Here is the image of the classic halo braid.

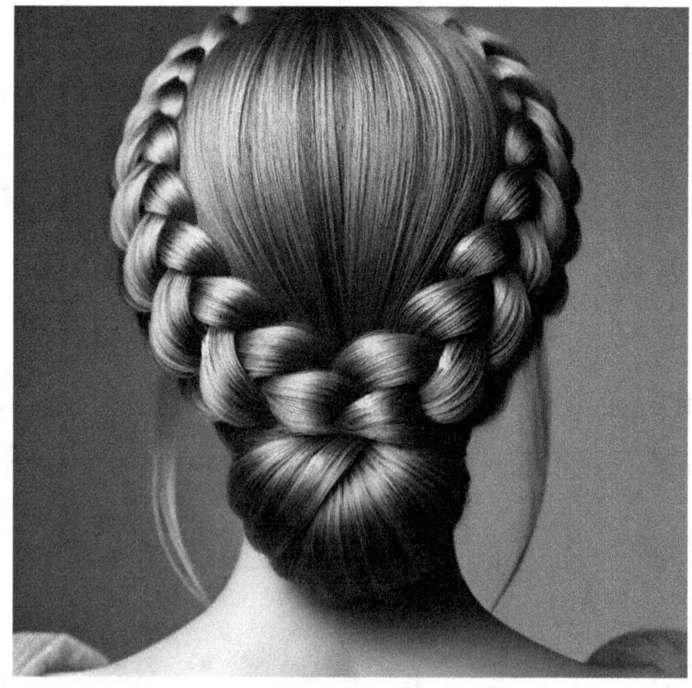

Instructions:

Step 1. Prep the Hair:

Detangle and smooth the hair with a brush. For extra volume, use a texturizing spray or dry shampoo to give the braid more grip and body.

Step 2. Part the Hair:

Part the hair in the center or slightly off-center, depending on your preference. This part will help guide the braid's direction.

Step 3. Start Braiding Near the Nape:

Begin by taking three sections of hair from near the nape of the neck, close to one ear. Start a Dutch braid (crossing the sections under the middle) or a French braid (crossing the sections over the middle).

- Braid along the hairline, adding sections of hair from both sides as you work your way up and around the head.

Step 4. Braid Around the Head:

Continue braiding around the head in a circular motion. Make sure to add hair from both sides evenly to maintain balance.

- Keep the braid snug but not too tight, as the goal is for it to sit softly on top of the head.

Step 5. Finish the Braid:

Once you have braided all the way around and used up the loose hair, continue with a simple three-strand braid at the end.

- Tuck the end of the braid under the starting point and secure it with bobby pins.

Step 6. Loosen and Adjust:

Gently pull on the edges of the braid to pancake it, creating a fuller, more voluminous appearance.

- Adjust the braid so that it sits evenly on top of the head, resembling a halo.

Styling Tips:

- Textured Halo: Add texture by using a curling iron to create waves before starting the braid. This adds softness and volume.

- Face-Framing Strands: Leave a few face-framing strands loose around the hairline for a more casual, romantic look.

- Accessorize: Adorn the braid with small flowers, pearls, or jeweled hairpins to enhance its angelic appearance.

2. Dutch Halo Braid

The Dutch halo braid is a bolder, raised version of the halo braid, created using the Dutch braiding technique (crossing strands under the middle section). This style stands out more from the head and has a more defined, textured appearance.

Here is the image of the Dutch halo braid.

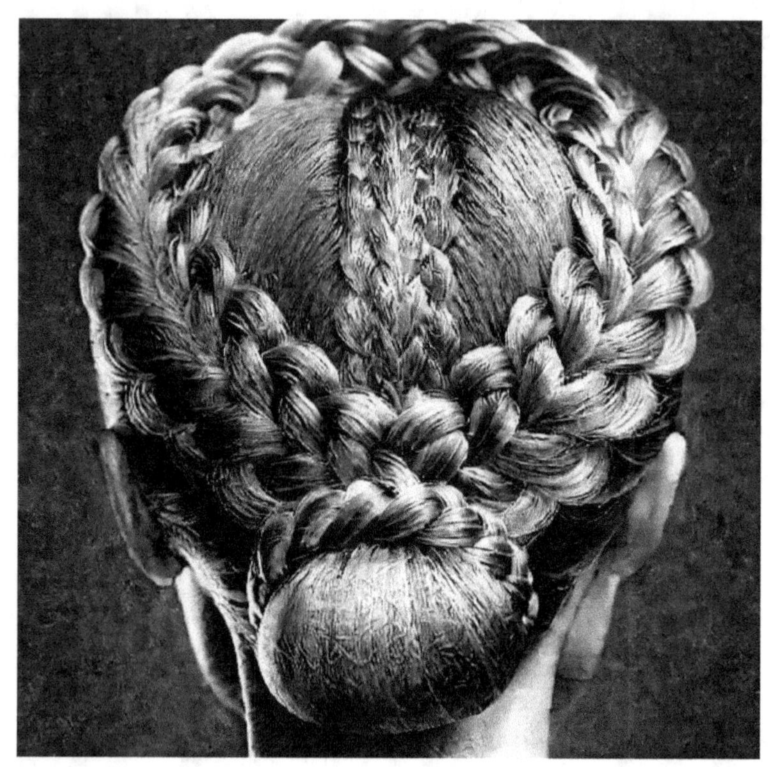

Instructions:

Step 1. Prep and Part:

Detangle the hair and apply a texturizing spray for volume. Part the hair in the center or off to the side, depending on the look you want.

Step 2. Start with a Dutch Braid:

Start near the nape of the neck, taking three small sections and beginning a Dutch braid. The key difference in this braid is that you will cross the strands under the middle section, making the braid stand out from the head.

Step 3. Braid Around the Head:

Continue the Dutch braid around the head, adding sections from both sides as you go. Keep the braid tight and close to the scalp to maintain its shape.

- Make sure to braid evenly around the hairline to create a consistent circular shape.

Step 4. Finish and Tuck:

Once you reach the starting point, finish with a regular three-strand braid. Tuck the end of the braid underneath the beginning and secure it with bobby pins.

- If needed, add extra pins to keep the braid secure and in place.

Step 5. Pancake the Braid:

Gently pull on the edges of the braid to widen it and give it a fuller, more voluminous look. The pancaking will also enhance the raised appearance of the Dutch braid.

Styling Tips:

- Volume Boost: Use a volumizing mousse or root-lifting spray before braiding to give the braid extra height and texture.
- Boho Style: For a more bohemian look, pull out a few strands along the hairline to create a slightly messy, undone effect.
- Statement Accessories: Add a statement headband or hairpiece at the front to give the Dutch halo braid a more dramatic look.

3. Fishtail Halo Braid

For a more intricate and detailed look, the fishtail halo braid is a beautiful variation that uses the fishtail braiding technique to create a more textured, woven appearance. This style is perfect for special occasions and adds a unique twist to the traditional halo braid.

Here is the image of the fishtail halo braid.

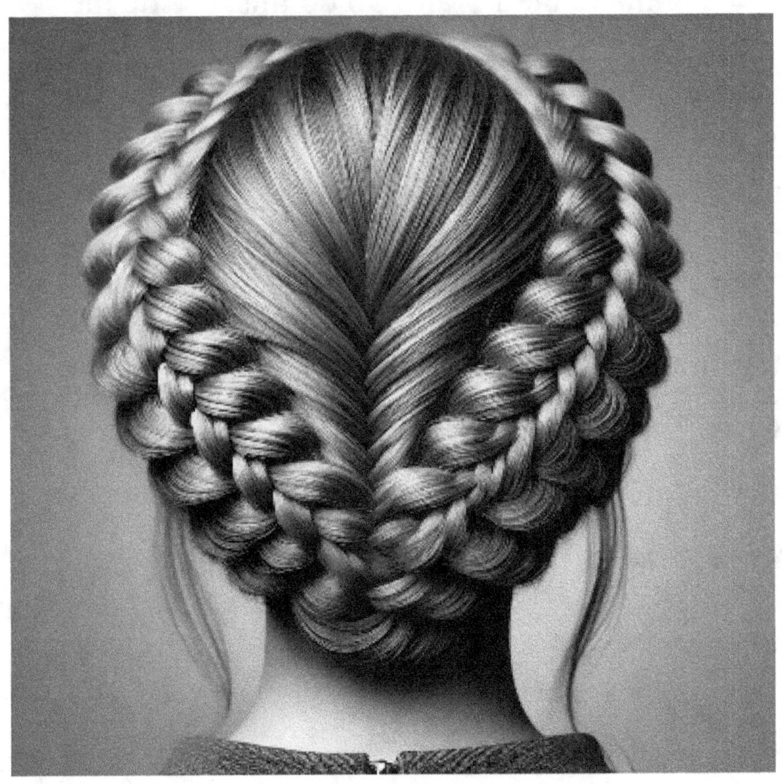

Instructions:

Step 1. Prep the Hair:

Detangle and smooth the hair, then divide it into two sections. Use a texturizing spray for added grip, especially if you have fine or slippery hair.

Step 2. Start the Fishtail Braid:

Take a small section of hair near the ear or nape and begin a fishtail braid. To do this, divide the section into two parts and take small strands from the outer edge of each section, crossing them over to the opposite side.

Step 3. Braid Around the Head:

Continue the fishtail braid along the hairline, working around the head in a circular pattern. Be sure to pick up small sections of hair as you go to incorporate them into the braid.

- Keep the braid snug but not too tight, as fishtail braids look best when slightly loosened.

Step 4. Complete the Braid:

Once you've braided around the head, finish with a regular fishtail braid. Secure the end with an elastic, then tuck it under the starting point and pin it in place.

Step 5. Loosen the Fishtail Braid:

Gently tug on the edges of the braid to pancake it and give it a more voluminous, airy appearance. This will also enhance the intricate fishtail pattern.

Styling Tips:

- Boho-Chic: For a relaxed, bohemian style, leave a few face-framing pieces loose and gently tousle the braid for a more laid-back look.

- Detailed Finish: The fishtail braid itself is highly detailed, so keep the overall look soft and natural to highlight the intricate braiding technique.

- Flowers or Accessories: Enhance the fishtail halo braid by pinning small flowers or embellishments into the braid, perfect for weddings or summer events.

4. Half-Up Halo Braid

If you prefer to leave some of your hair down, the half-up halo braid is a great alternative. This style features a braid around the top half of the head, while the rest of the hair is left loose, creating a blend of structure and flow.

Here is the image of the half-up halo braid.

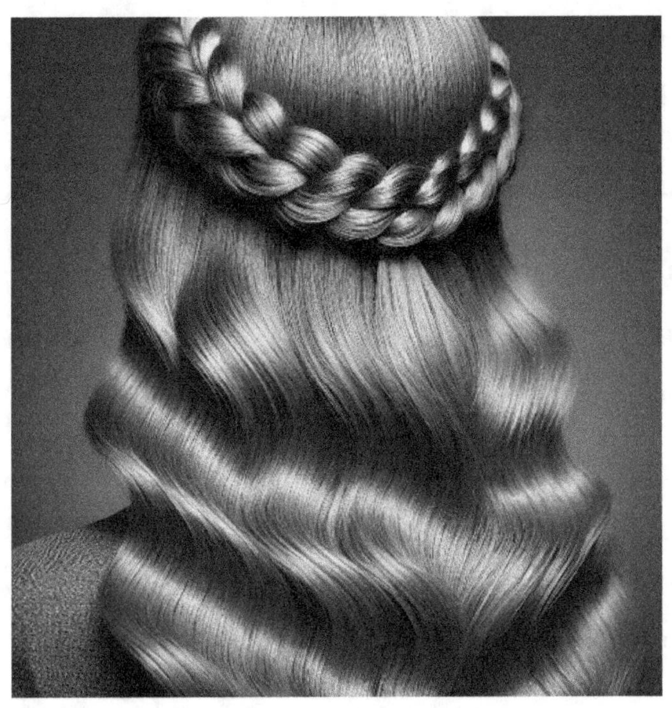

Instructions:

Step 1. Part the Hair and Section:

Part the hair down the middle or to the side, then section off the top half of your hair, leaving the bottom half loose.

Step 2. Start the Braid:

Begin braiding near one ear, either using a Dutch or French braid. Work your way around the crown of the head, incorporating small sections of hair as you go.

Step 3. Braid Around the Crown:

Continue braiding until you reach the opposite ear. Secure the braid with a small elastic and tuck the end underneath the braid, pinning it securely.

Step 4. Style the Loose Hair:

For a cohesive look, curl or wave the loose sections of hair to add texture and volume.

Step 5. Loosen the Braid:

Gently pull on the edges of the braid to pancake it, making it look fuller and more relaxed.

Styling Tips:

- Casual Look: For a more casual, everyday look, keep the braid tight and the loose hair straight or slightly tousled.

- Formal Finish: For a more polished finish, curl the loose hair and add hair accessories like a headband or flowers to the braid.

The halo braid is an incredibly versatile hairstyle that can be customized to suit any occasion, from casual days to formal events. Whether you prefer a simple, classic halo braid, a bold Dutch halo braid, or a more intricate fishtail halo braid, this style is both elegant and practical. With the right technique and a few finishing touches, you can create a stunning, angelic look that is sure to turn heads.

3. Waterfall Braids: The Elegant, Cascading Style

The waterfall braid is a romantic and intricate braiding technique that creates a cascading effect by "dropping" sections of hair through the braid, resembling a waterfall. This braid is perfect for adding elegance to loose hairstyles and works beautifully for both casual and formal occasions. It pairs especially well with wavy or curly hair, giving the overall style a soft, flowing look.

1. Classic Waterfall Braid

The classic waterfall braid begins with a French braiding technique but differs in that the lower sections of the braid are "dropped" or released, creating a cascading waterfall effect. This braid works well on medium to long hair and is ideal for half-up, half-down styles.

Here is the colored image of a classic waterfall braid.

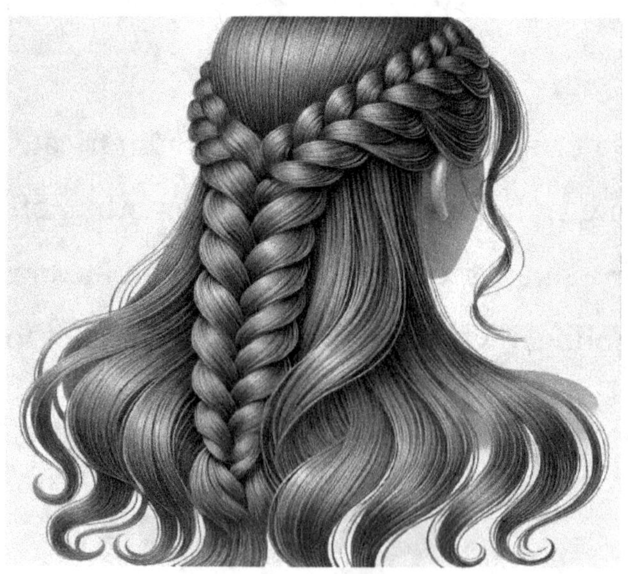

Instructions:

Step 1. Part the Hair:

Start with a side part or center part, depending on where you want the braid to flow. Brush your hair to remove any tangles and make the braiding process smoother.

Step 2. Start a French Braid:

Take a section of hair near your temple (on one side) and divide it into three equal parts.

Begin braiding as you would a normal French braid, crossing the top section over the middle, followed by the bottom section over the middle.

Step 3. Drop the Bottom Section:

After the first couple of passes, instead of incorporating the bottom section into the braid, drop it and let it fall naturally. This is what creates the waterfall effect.

Step 4. Replace the Dropped Section:

Pick up a new section of hair directly behind the dropped section to replace it. Cross this new section over the middle strand and continue braiding.

Step 5. Continue the Waterfall Pattern:

Repeat the process: drop the bottom section, pick up a new piece of hair, and continue French braiding. Keep this pattern going as you braid horizontally across the back of your head.

Step 6. Secure the Braid:

Once you've braided as far as you want (usually to the opposite side of the head), you can either pin the braid with bobby pins for a half-up style or continue with a simple three-strand braid down the remaining length of hair. Secure with an elastic.

Step 7. Adjust the Braid:

Gently pull on the braid to loosen it and create a fuller, softer look. If needed, use bobby pins to secure any loose strands.

Styling Tips:

- Waves and Curls: The waterfall braid looks especially beautiful when combined with wavy or curly hair. You can create soft waves with a curling iron before braiding for a more romantic, textured style.
- Pancaking: For a more voluminous look, gently tug on the braid's edges (pancaking) to make it appear fuller and more relaxed.

2. Double Waterfall Braid

The double waterfall braid takes the classic waterfall braid to the next level by adding a second braid directly below the first, creating a layered, intricate effect. This style is ideal for long hair and special occasions where you want an extra touch of elegance.

Here is the image of a double waterfall braid.

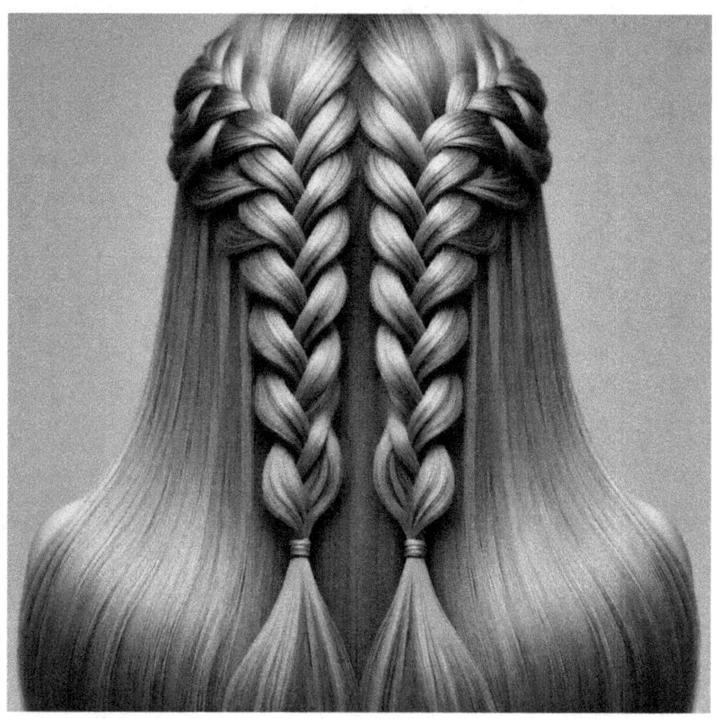

Instructions:

Step 1. Create the First Waterfall Braid:

Follow the steps for a classic waterfall braid, starting near the temple and braiding across the back of the head. Drop sections as you go, and continue until you reach the opposite side.

Step 2. Start the Second Waterfall Braid:

After finishing the first braid, begin the second waterfall braid directly below the first one. Use the dropped sections from the first braid as part of the new braid.

- Pick up hair from the dropped sections and new sections from below to incorporate into the second braid.

Step 3. Braid Across and Secure:

Continue braiding the second waterfall braid in the same direction as the first. Secure the end of the braid with bobby pins or an elastic once you've completed it.

Step 4. Finish with Loose Hair or a Braid:

For a half-up style, leave the rest of your hair loose. You can also gather the remaining hair into a simple braid or fishtail braid for added texture.

Styling Tips:

- Layered Look: This style is perfect for adding dimension to layered haircuts, as the different lengths of hair create more texture and movement.
- Subtle Twists: For a twist on the classic, try twisting the waterfall sections before dropping them to add a more intricate detail.

3. Waterfall Braid into a Fishtail Braid

For a more intricate, hybrid style, the waterfall braid into a fishtail braid combines the delicate waterfall technique with the beautiful complexity of a fishtail braid. This is an ideal hairstyle for long hair and formal events like weddings or proms.

Here is the image of the hairstyle transitioning from a waterfall braid into a fishtail braid.

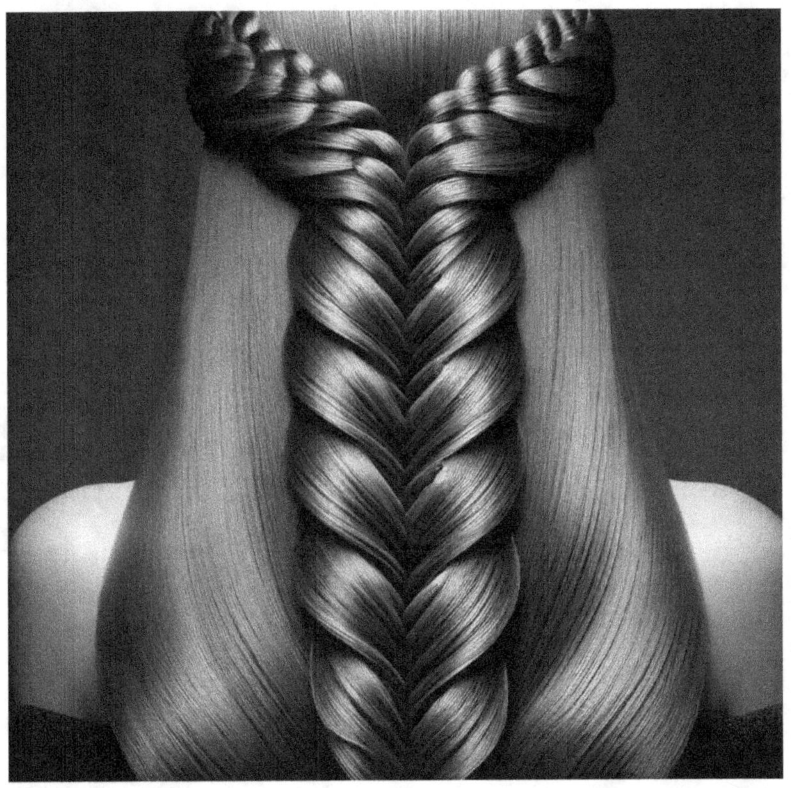

Instructions:

Step 1. Start with a Waterfall Braid:

Begin with a classic waterfall braid by braiding from one side of your head to the other, dropping sections as you go and picking up new ones. Braid

across the back of your head until you reach the
other side.

Step 2. Gather the Remaining Hair:

Once you've finished the waterfall braid, gather all
the remaining hair (including the dropped sections)
into a low ponytail at the nape of your neck.

Step 3. Start a Fishtail Braid:

Divide the ponytail into two sections. Begin a
fishtail braid by taking small strands from the outer
edge of each section and crossing them over to the
opposite section.

- Continue braiding down the length of the
  hair.

Step 4. Secure and Adjust:

Once you've finished the fishtail braid, secure the
end with a small elastic. For added texture and
volume, gently pancake the fishtail braid by
tugging on the edges.

Step 5. Blend the Waterfall with the Fishtail:

Make sure the transition between the waterfall braid and the fishtail braid is smooth and seamless. You can add a decorative hairpin or ribbon where the two braids meet to enhance the look.

Styling Tips:

- Romantic Waves: To make this style even more romantic, curl the loose sections of the waterfall braid before incorporating them into the fishtail braid.
- Accessorize: Add a few small flowers, beads, or pearl pins throughout the waterfall and fishtail braid for a fairytale-inspired look.

4. Waterfall Crown Braid

The waterfall crown braid is a sophisticated, circular braid that wraps around the head, resembling a crown. It combines the elegance of the waterfall technique with the structure of a crown braid, making it a perfect choice for formal events like weddings or galas.

Here is the image of the waterfall crown braid.

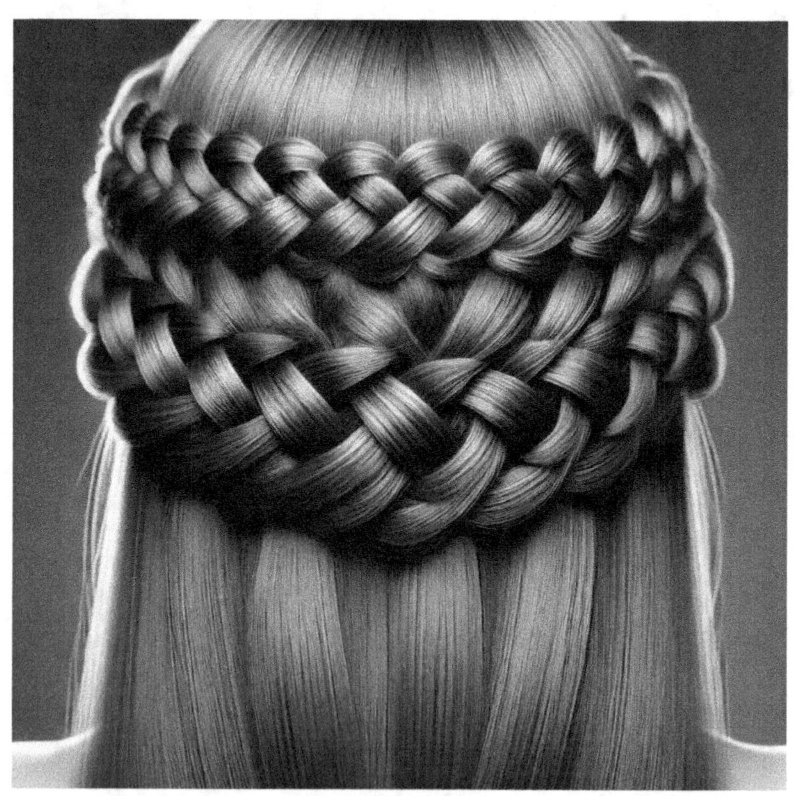

Instructions:

Step 1. Part and Section the Hair:

Part the hair down the middle or to one side, depending on your preference. Take a section of hair near the temple to start the waterfall braid.

Step 2. Begin the Waterfall Braid:

Start braiding around the perimeter of the head, using the waterfall braid technique. Drop sections as you go, letting them fall naturally, and pick up new sections to continue the braid.

Step 3. Continue Around the Head:

Braid in a circular motion around the head, following the hairline. Continue dropping sections and replacing them as you go. The braid should wrap around your head like a crown.

Note: you can choose to braid around the head twice to have more intricate design.

Step 4. Tuck and Pin:

Once you've finished braiding around the entire head, secure the end of the braid by tucking it under the starting point and pinning it with bobby pins.

Step 5. Loosen for Volume:

Gently pull on the braid's edges to make it appear fuller and softer. The dropped sections will cascade like a waterfall, creating a beautiful crown effect.

Styling Tips:

- Royal Accessories: Add jeweled hairpins or small flowers around the braid for a more formal, bridal look.
- Half-Up, Half-Down: You can combine this braid with loose curls or waves for a stunning half-up, half-down hairstyle that balances structure and flow.

The waterfall braid is a versatile and elegant style that offers endless possibilities for creativity. Whether you prefer the classic waterfall braid, the double waterfall braid, or a hybrid style like the waterfall braid into a fishtail, this technique adds a delicate, cascading effect to any hairstyle. Perfect for weddings, proms, or everyday wear, waterfall braids are an excellent way to showcase your braiding skills while adding softness and romance to your look.

4. Braided Flower Buns: A Beautiful Floral-Inspired Hair Design

The braided flower bun is an intricate and eye-catching hairstyle that resembles the shape of a blooming flower. This style is perfect for formal events, weddings, or any occasion where you want to create a memorable look. By combining basic braiding techniques with clever twists and coils, you can create a bun that looks like a flower, adding elegance and creativity to your style.

1. Simple Braided Flower Bun

The simple braided flower bun starts with a regular braid or fishtail braid that is coiled into a bun, forming the petals of a flower. The wider and looser the braid, the more pronounced the "petals" appear, creating a floral effect.

Here is the image of the simple braided flower bun.

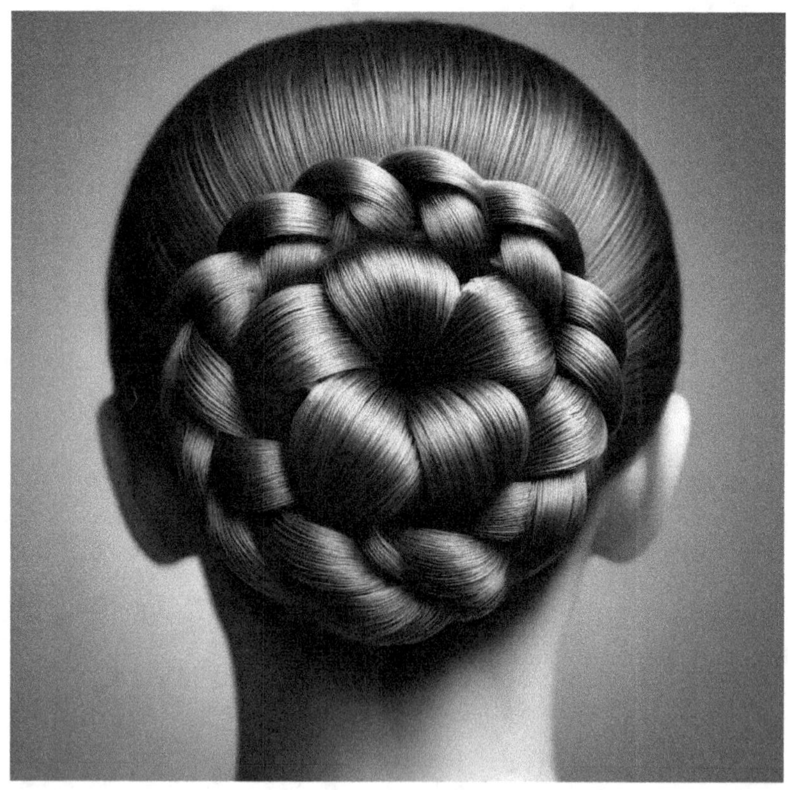

Instructions:

Step 1. Prep the Hair:

Start by brushing your hair to remove any tangles. You can also apply a smoothing serum to give the braid a sleek, polished look.

Step 2. Create a Ponytail:

Gather your hair into a low or high ponytail, depending on where you want the flower bun to sit (at the nape of the neck or higher on the crown). Secure the ponytail with a hair tie.

Step 3. Braid the Ponytail:

Divide the ponytail into three sections and create a simple three-strand braid. Braid down the length of the ponytail, keeping the tension even. Secure the end with a small elastic band.

Step 4. Pancake the Braid:

To create the petals of the flower, gently pull on the edges of the braid (called pancaking) to loosen and widen it. The braid should look fuller and softer, giving it a petal-like appearance.

Step 5. Coil the Braid into a Bun:

Starting at the base of the ponytail, coil the braided ponytail around itself in a circular motion to form the bun. The pancaked sections of the braid will mimic the look of flower petals.

Step 6. Secure the Bun:

Pin the bun in place using bobby pins, making sure to hide the ends of the braid underneath the bun for a seamless finish.

Step 7. Finishing Touches:

Use hairspray to smooth any flyaways and ensure the bun stays secure throughout the day.

Styling Tips:

- Add Texture: If you want a more bohemian or textured look, start with slightly wavy hair or add a texturizing spray before braiding.

- Decorate with Accessories: Enhance the flower-like appearance by adding small flowers, jeweled pins, or pearls around the bun.

2. Fishtail Braided Flower Bun

The fishtail braided flower bun adds an extra level of intricacy by using the fishtail braiding technique. The fine, woven look of the fishtail braid makes the flower bun appear more detailed and delicate, perfect for formal events like weddings or galas.

Here is the image of the fishtail braided flower bun.

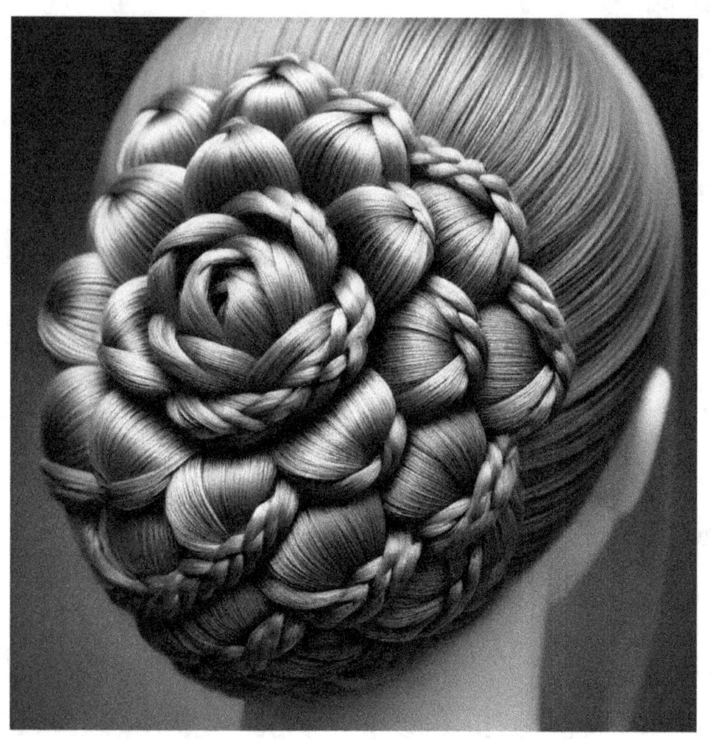

Instructions:

Step 1. Create a Fishtail Braid:

Start by gathering your hair into a ponytail and secure it with a hair tie.

- Divide the ponytail into two sections and begin a fishtail braid by taking a small strand of hair from the outer edge of one section and crossing it over to the other section. Repeat this on the opposite side and continue braiding down the length of the ponytail.

Step 2. Pancake the Fishtail Braid:

Gently pull on the edges of the fishtail braid to widen it and give it more volume. This will create a softer, more petal-like appearance.

Step 3. Coil the Braid into a Bun:

Starting at the base of the ponytail, carefully coil the fishtail braid around itself to form a bun. The pancaked fishtail braid will resemble flower petals as you coil it in a circular shape.

Step 4. Secure with Bobby Pins:

Use bobby pins to secure the bun in place. Make sure to hide the ends of the braid by tucking them underneath the bun.

Step 5. Refine the Look:

Adjust the bun to ensure it looks symmetrical and flower-like. Pull gently on the edges if you need to create more volume. Use hairspray to keep everything in place.

Styling Tips:

- Boho Vibe: For a relaxed, boho look, leave a few face-framing strands loose around the hairline.
- Accessories: Place small decorative pins or flowers around the bun for an ethereal, nature-inspired finish.

3. Double Braided Flower Bun

For a more intricate and voluminous look, you can create a double braided flower bun by combining two braids into one floral-inspired bun. This style is perfect for long, thick hair and adds extra dimension to the flower shape.

Here is the image of the double braided flower bun.

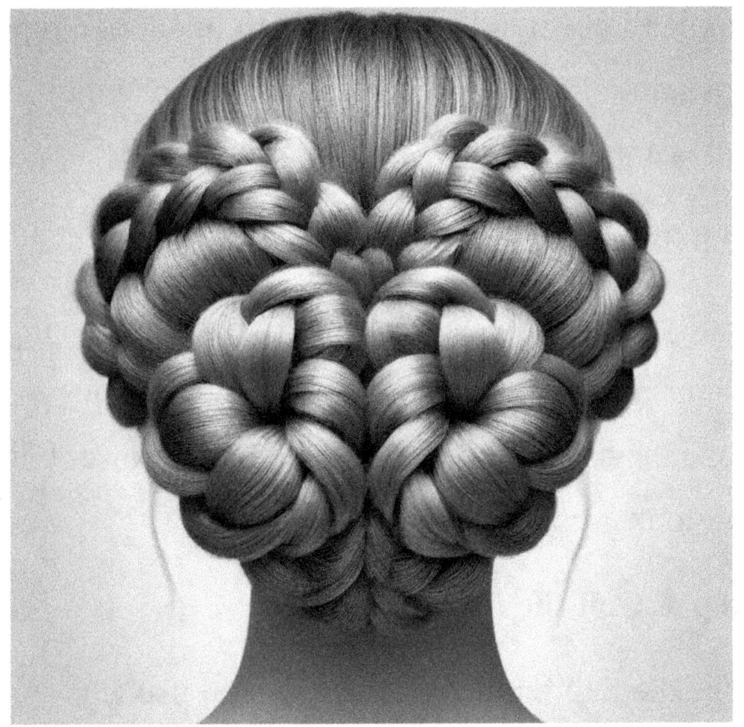

Instructions:

Step 1. Divide the Hair into Two Sections:

Start by dividing your hair into two equal sections. You can part it down the middle or slightly off-center, depending on where you want the buns to sit.

Step 2. Create Two Braids:

Braid each section separately. You can use a simple three-strand braid, a fishtail braid, or a rope twist braid for added texture. Secure each braid with a small elastic.

Step 3. Pancake Both Braids:

Gently pull on the edges of both braids to widen them, creating the petal effect. The wider you make the braids, the more dramatic the flower bun will look.

Step 4. Coil the First Braid:

Take the first braid and coil it around itself, forming a bun. Secure the bun with bobby pins.

Step 5. Add the Second Braid:

Take the second braid and coil it around the first bun, creating a layered, flower-like effect. Secure with bobby pins.

Step 6. Adjust and Secure:

Adjust both braids to ensure the bun looks even and symmetrical. Use more bobby pins to secure any loose strands and keep the bun in place.

Styling Tips:

- Layered Braids: Use two different types of braids (e.g., one three-strand braid and one fishtail braid) to create more texture and dimension.
- Formal Elegance: For a formal look, keep the braids sleek and polished. For a more relaxed vibe, allow a few pieces of hair to remain loose and tousled.

4. Flower Bun with Twisted Accents

For an extra touch of detail, you can combine a braided flower bun with twisted sections of hair. The twists add additional texture and complexity to the style, making it look even more like a blooming flower.

Here is the image of the flower bun with twisted accents.

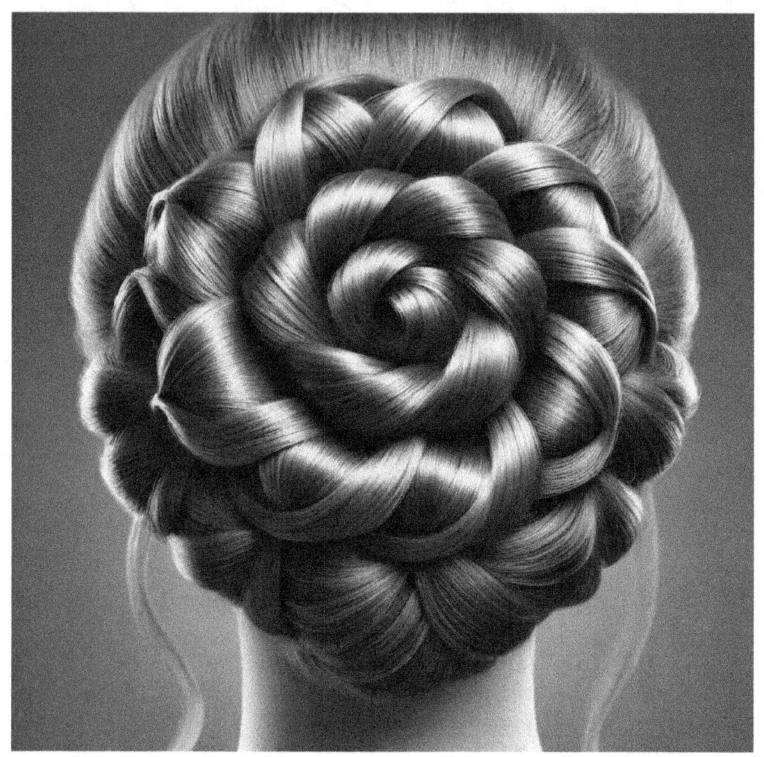

Instructions:

Step 1. Section the Hair:

Divide your hair into three sections: one large section in the back for the bun and two smaller sections on either side for the twists.

Step 2. Create the Braided Bun:

Gather the large back section into a ponytail and create a three-strand braid or fishtail braid. Pancake the braid for volume and coil it into a bun, securing it with bobby pins.

Step 3. Add Twisted Sections:

Take the two smaller sections on either side of your head and twist them toward the back. Wrap each twisted section around the bun and pin them in place.

Step 4. Secure and Adjust:

Use bobby pins to secure the twisted sections, tucking the ends underneath the bun. Adjust the bun and twists to ensure the style looks full and symmetrical.

Step 5. Finishing Touches:

Use hairspray to set the style and tame any flyaways. Add small hair accessories or decorative pins to the bun or twists for an extra touch of elegance.

Styling Tips:

- Twist Variations: Try incorporating small braids into the twists for added texture and detail.
- Loose and Flowing: For a softer look, leave the twisted sections slightly loose and allow some tendrils to fall naturally around your face.

Braided flower buns are a stunning way to elevate any look, combining the elegance of braids with the artistry of floral shapes. Whether you opt for a simple braided bun, a fishtail flower bun, or a more intricate double flower bun, these styles are perfect for formal occasions, weddings, or any event where you want to stand out. With a bit of practice, these braided buns can become a go-to style for adding a touch of creativity and sophistication to your hair.

Chapter 7

Combining Braids for More Complex Designs

Once you've mastered basic braiding techniques like the three-strand, French, Dutch, and fishtail braids, you can start combining them to create more intricate, visually stunning styles. These combined braids are perfect for special occasions or when you want to elevate your everyday look. Here's how to layer, blend, and merge different braiding styles to design complex, multi-dimensional hairstyles.

1. Combination of French Braid and Fishtail Braid

This style combines the neatness and scalp-hugging structure of the French braid with the intricate, delicate detail of the fishtail braid. You can start with a French braid at the crown of the head and transition into a fishtail braid as you move toward the ends.

Instructions:

Step 1. Start with a French Braid:

Begin by sectioning a portion of hair from the crown and divide it into three sections for a French braid.

- As you braid, add hair from the sides of your head until you reach the nape of the neck.

Step 2. Transition into a Fishtail Braid:

Once you have braided down to the nape and all hair is incorporated into the French braid, stop adding new sections.

- Divide the remaining hair into two sections and switch to a fishtail braid by taking small strands from each side and crossing them over to the opposite side.

Step 3. Finish and Secure:

Continue the fishtail braid until you reach the ends of your hair and secure it with an elastic. The

transition from French braid to fishtail gives a
smooth and elegant look with increased texture
and complexity toward the bottom.

Key Tips:

- Tightness Control: Keep the French braid
  tight near the scalp to anchor the style, then
  slightly loosen the fishtail braid for a more
  relaxed, flowing effect.
- Smooth Transition: When switching from
  French to fishtail, ensure the sectioning is
  even, so the transition looks natural.

2. Dutch Braid into a Crown Braid with Fishtail Accents

In this design, a Dutch braid is woven into a crown
braid, and the ends of the hair are styled into
fishtail braid accents for extra detail and texture.
This style gives the appearance of a halo or crown
around the head, with intricate detailing.

Instructions:

Step 1. Create the Dutch Braid Crown:

- Part your hair slightly off-center and begin with a Dutch braid on one side of the head.
- Braid along the perimeter of your hairline, adding sections as you go.
- Continue braiding around the head until you complete a full circle and meet at the starting point.

Step 2. Tuck and Secure the Crown:

Once you've finished the Dutch braid, tuck the end of the braid under the starting point and secure it with bobby pins. This forms the base of the crown braid.

Step 3. Add Fishtail Braid Accents:

- Take the remaining hair from the ends of the Dutch braid or any loose hair and create small fishtail braids.

- Wrap these fishtail braids around the crown braid, pinning them in place to add texture and depth.

Step 4. Secure and Finish:

Use bobby pins to secure the fishtail braids. Gently loosen the fishtail sections to give the look a fuller, more textured appearance.

Key Tips:

- Balance the Braids: Make sure the Dutch braid is evenly sized around the head for a balanced crown shape. Loosen it slightly for a softer, more romantic look.
- Highlight the Fishtail: Pancake (pull gently on the fishtail braid's edges) to make it stand out and give it a textured, voluminous effect.

3. Double Braided Headband with a Fishtail Ponytail

This style uses two thin Dutch braids along the top of the head, creating a headband effect. These braids transition into a fishtail ponytail at the back for a chic, modern look.

Instructions:

Step 1. Part the Hair and Start Two Thin Dutch Braids:

Part the hair down the middle. On each side, start small Dutch braids near the front of your hairline, working back toward the crown.

- Continue Dutch braiding down to the nape, leaving the rest of the hair loose.

Step 2. Combine the Dutch Braids into a Ponytail:

Once the two Dutch braids meet at the back, gather the remaining hair, including the loose sections, into a ponytail.

- Secure the ponytail with an elastic.

Step 3. Create the Fishtail Braid:

Divide the ponytail into two sections and begin a fishtail braid.

- Continue braiding the ponytail until you reach the ends, then secure with a small hair tie.

Step 4. Loosen the Braids for Volume:

Gently pull apart the two Dutch braids and the fishtail braid to give them more volume and texture.

Key Tips:

- Neatness with Dutch Braids: Keep the Dutch braids tight along the scalp to create a clean headband effect. The contrast between the tight Dutch braids and the looser fishtail braid adds dimension.
- Styling Options: This style works well with accessories like hairpins or flowers to accent the braids.

4. Waterfall Braid Merging into a Fishtail or Three-Strand Braid

The waterfall braid is a beautiful, flowing braid that leaves strands of hair cascading down, giving it a romantic look. Combine it with a fishtail braid or a three-strand braid at the back for added complexity and texture.

Instructions:

Step 1. Start with a Waterfall Braid:

Take a section of hair at the front and begin a regular French braid, but instead of pulling all the hair into the braid, drop the bottom section after crossing it over. This creates a "waterfall" effect as strands are left out to fall naturally.

- Continue this pattern across the head, dropping sections of hair and incorporating new ones into the braid.

Step 2. Transition into a Fishtail or Three-Strand Braid:

Once the waterfall braid reaches the back of the head, gather all the loose sections along with the braid and divide them into two for a fishtail braid or three for a classic three-strand braid.

- Continue braiding down the length of the hair and secure the braid with an elastic.

Step 3. Final Touches:

Loosen the waterfall braid slightly to give it a softer, more romantic look.

- For added texture, gently pancake the fishtail braid or leave the three-strand braid tight for a more polished appearance.

Key Tips:

- Perfect the Waterfall Braid: Practice keeping the waterfall sections even, as this will create a balanced look.

- Soft vs. Tight Finish: You can decide whether to keep the final braid (fishtail or three-strand) tight for a sleek look or loose for a more casual vibe.

5. Braided Bun with Twisted Accents

This style combines a three-strand braid or Dutch braid with twisted sections to create a voluminous braided bun, perfect for formal occasions. Twisted accents add texture and dimension around the bun.

Instructions:

Step 1. Create a Braid:

Start with a basic three-strand braid or Dutch braid from the nape of the neck, working your way down.

Step 2. Form the Bun:

Once the braid is complete, wrap it into a bun at the back of your head, securing it with bobby pins.

Step 3. Add Twisted Accents:

Take smaller sections of hair from around the face or sides and twist them. Secure the twists by pinning them into the base of the bun for added detail.

Step 4. Secure and Style:

Pin the bun securely and finish with hairspray to keep everything in place.

Key Tips:

- Tight or Loose Braid: Depending on the occasion, keep the braid tight for a more formal, polished bun or loosen it for a casual, boho-inspired look.
- Twist Variation: You can also create small fishtail braids for the twisted accents instead of simple twists for a more intricate design.

Note: Combining braiding techniques opens the door to creating unique, complex hairstyles that can elevate your look for any occasion. By along the braid's edges for a soft, floral look.

- Individual Flower Pins: Pin individual flowers sporadically throughout a fishtail braid, waterfall braid, or flower bun to mimic a blooming garden.
- Floral Headbands: For a bold statement, use a pre-made floral crown or headband and place it around the base of your braid, securing it with bobby pins if needed.

Styling Tips:

- Fresh Flowers: Keep fresh flowers in water until you're ready to use them to avoid wilting. For longer-lasting styles, opt for dried flowers or high-quality silk flowers.
- Minimalist Approach: Use just a few strategically placed flowers for a subtle, elegant look, or go all out with a full floral crown for a more dramatic, festival-ready style.

2. Ribbons and Threads

Adding ribbons or colored threads to braids can create a whimsical, colorful effect. This is great for casual looks, themed events, or adding a pop of color to your hair.

How to Use:

- Weave a Ribbon Through the Braid: Starting at the base of your braid, weave a thin ribbon through each strand as you braid. This works well with three-strand or fishtail braids.
- Braid with Thread: For smaller accents, you can braid colored embroidery thread into the sections of your braid, allowing the thread to peek through the braid for a subtle touch of color.
- Ribbon Bows: Tie a small ribbon bow at the end of your braid to secure it, adding a feminine touch.

Tips for All Hair Types

Avoid Tight Braids: No matter your hair type, avoid pulling the hair too tightly when braiding, as it can lead to scalp discomfort, tension headaches, and even hair loss.

Use a Satin or Silk Scarf: To maintain braids overnight and reduce frizz, wrap your braids in a satin or silk scarf, or sleep on a satin pillowcase.

Keep the Scalp Moisturized: Especially with protective styles like box braids or cornrows, keeping the scalp hydrated is essential. Use lightweight oils like jojoba or argan oil to keep the scalp healthy without causing buildup.

Finish with Hairspray or Serum: For extra hold, use a light mist of hairspray to set the braids in place. A shine serum can also be applied to give the braids a sleek, polished finish.

Note: Braiding is versatile and can be adapted to all hair types and textures. Whether you have fine,

2. Ribbons and Threads

Adding ribbons or colored threads to braids can create a whimsical, colorful effect. This is great for casual looks, themed events, or adding a pop of color to your hair.

How to Use:

- Weave a Ribbon Through the Braid: Starting at the base of your braid, weave a thin ribbon through each strand as you braid. This works well with three-strand or fishtail braids.
- Braid with Thread: For smaller accents, you can braid colored embroidery thread into the sections of your braid, allowing the thread to peek through the braid for a subtle touch of color.
- Ribbon Bows: Tie a small ribbon bow at the end of your braid to secure it, adding a feminine touch.

Styling Tips:

- Contrast or Match: Use contrasting colors (like gold or vibrant hues) to make the ribbon stand out, or choose a ribbon that matches your hair color for a more subtle effect.
- Bohemian Vibes: Combine ribbon or thread with a loose, messy braid for a boho-chic look that's great for festivals or beach days.

3. Beads and Charms

Adding beads or charms to your braids brings texture and personality to the style. This is especially popular for bohemian looks, festival styles, or to add a cultural element to your hair.

How to Use:

- Beads on Box Braids or Cornrows: Add wooden or metallic beads to the ends of box braids or cornrows for a classic, bohemian look. Use a beading tool or a small elastic to secure the beads in place.

- Charms: Clip or tie small charms (like stars, shells, or moons) throughout the length of a fishtail or three-strand braid for a fun, celestial effect.

- Beads Threaded Into Braids: Thread beads onto a thin string and braid them into the hair, letting the beads sit sporadically throughout the braid.

Styling Tips:

- Minimalist Approach: Use just a few beads or charms for a subtle, modern look.

- Statement Look: For a more striking style, you can fill the ends of braids with multiple beads in different sizes and materials (wood, metal, or plastic) for a cultural-inspired design.

4. Hair Chains and Jewelry

Hair chains and jewelry add an element of luxury and sophistication to your braids, making them ideal for formal events, weddings, or glamorous parties.

How to Use:

- Drape Chains Over Braids: Drape delicate chains across the top of a crown braid or halo braid. Secure the chains with bobby pins at the beginning and end of the braid.
- Clip-In Jewelry: Clip-in jewelry pieces (like crystal-encrusted combs or metallic headpieces) can be placed at the sides or top of braided styles like French braids or flower buns.
- Embellished Pins: Use rhinestone or pearl-embellished pins and place them at intervals along the braid to add sparkle and elegance.

Styling Tips:

- Go for Gold or Silver: Metallic hair chains in gold or silver can complement your jewelry or outfit, adding a cohesive, sophisticated look.
- Layer the Chains: For a bolder look, layer multiple chains or mix metals (gold, rose gold, and silver) for a dynamic and stylish effect.

5. Hair Rings and Cuffs

Hair rings and cuffs are a bold and edgy way to accessorize braids. This trend has gained popularity in festival fashion and street style for its modern, warrior-like aesthetic.

How to Use:

- Hair Rings in Cornrows or Box Braids: Open small metal hair rings and place them through sections of your cornrows or box braids for a stylish, edgy touch.

- Cuffs in Three-Strand or Dutch Braids: Slip small hair cuffs around sections of the braid, securing them in place along the braid's length.

- Mix and Match: Combine different sizes and styles of rings and cuffs throughout a single braid for a more eclectic look.

Styling Tips:

- Strategic Placement: Place rings or cuffs near the crown or middle of the braid to draw attention to the detail.

- Edgy Vibe: Combine this accessory with a tight Dutch braid or side braid for an edgy, bold look, perfect for concerts or festivals.

6. Pearls and Crystal Pins

Pearls and crystal pins give braids a refined and glamorous look. They're ideal for formal events, such as weddings, where you want to add a touch of sophistication and sparkle.

How to Use:

- Pearls in a Fishtail Braid: Pin small pearl hairpins sporadically through a fishtail braid or crown braid for an elegant, bridal-inspired look.

- Crystal Bobby Pins: Use crystal-encrusted bobby pins along the sides of a waterfall braid to add sparkle and keep loose strands in place.

- Pearl String Wrap: Wrap a string of pearls around a three-strand braid or flower bun, securing it with bobby pins to keep it in place.

Styling Tips:

- Subtle Glam: If you prefer a minimalist style, opt for just a few pearls or crystal pins scattered throughout the braid for a touch of glamour.

- Bridal Ready: For brides, using pearls or crystals can complement the wedding dress, creating a cohesive and elegant look that's perfect for the big day.

7. Scarves and Bandanas

Using scarves or bandanas in your braids adds texture, color, and a vintage or bohemian feel to your hairstyle. This is perfect for a casual day out, festivals, or when you want to add a pop of personality to your look.

How to Use:

- Braid a Scarf into Your Hair: Start with a small square scarf or bandana. Tie it around the base of your ponytail and incorporate it as a strand in a three-strand braid or Dutch braid.
- Wrap a Scarf Around a Bun: Tie a scarf around the base of a flower bun or braided bun for a retro-inspired look.

- Boho Bandana: Use a bandana as a headband and let your braids hang down beneath it for a casual, festival-ready style.

Styling Tips:

- Bohemian Style: Combine loose, messy braids with a scarf or bandana for a relaxed, boho-chic vibe.
- Bright Colors: Choose a scarf with bold colors or patterns to make a statement, or go with neutral tones for a more understated look.

Note: Adding accessories to your braids is a fantastic way to personalize and enhance your hairstyle, no matter the occasion. From delicate flowers and ribbons to hair rings, cuffs, and jewelry, there are endless ways to experiment with different materials and styles to suit your mood or event. Whether you're going for an elegant, boho, or edgy look, incorporating accessories into your braids will help you stand out with a unique and stunning hairstyle.

Chapter 9

Braiding for Different Hair Types and Textures

Braiding techniques can be adapted to suit different hair types and textures, whether your hair is fine and straight, wavy, curly, or coily. Each texture has unique characteristics, and knowing how to work with them can help you achieve neat, secure, and beautiful braids. Here's a guide to braiding techniques for various hair types, along with tips to ensure the best results.

1. Braiding Fine or Straight Hair

Characteristics:

Smooth and slippery: Fine hair tends to be sleek, which can make it difficult to hold braids securely without slipping.

Lack of volume: Fine hair can be flat and may not create as voluminous braids as other textures.

Braiding Techniques:

- Add Texture: Use a texturizing spray, mousse, or dry shampoo before braiding to give the hair more grip and body. This will help the braid stay in place and prevent it from slipping.

- Tight Braids: Braiding tightly will help prevent the strands from unraveling. Consider styles like a French braid or Dutch braid, which pull hair closer to the scalp and create a more secure hold.

- Tease the Hair for Volume: For added volume, gently backcomb or tease the sections of hair before braiding. This will make the braid look thicker and more substantial.

- Secure with Elastics: Always secure braids with small, clear elastics or hair ties to prevent them from loosening throughout the day.

Best Styles:

- Tight Dutch Braid: The underhand crossing technique adds dimension and gives the appearance of thicker hair.

- Double Braids or Pigtails: Dividing hair into two sections and braiding each side helps create the illusion of more volume.

- Fishtail Braid: The intricate weaving pattern of a fishtail braid adds texture and detail, making fine hair appear fuller.

2. Braiding Wavy Hair

Characteristics:

Natural texture: Wavy hair has a natural "S" shape that adds volume and movement to braids.

Frizz-prone: Wavy hair can become frizzy, especially in humid conditions.

Braiding Techniques:

- Embrace the Texture: Wavy hair naturally holds braids well, so you can take advantage of its volume and texture. Looser braids, like bohemian side braids or messy French braids, work beautifully with wavy hair.

- Moisturize to Prevent Frizz: Use a lightweight leave-in conditioner or anti-frizz serum before braiding to smooth the hair and keep the braid looking polished.

- Loose Braids for a Relaxed Look: Looser braids allow the natural waves to peek through, giving a soft, romantic vibe. A waterfall braid or loose fishtail braid can highlight the natural movement of wavy hair.

- Curl the Ends: If your waves don't extend all the way to the tips, consider curling the ends after braiding to blend the braid with the natural wave pattern.

Best Styles:

Boho Side Braid: A side braid with loose, pancaked edges gives a relaxed, flowing look.

Waterfall Braid: This style allows sections of wavy hair to cascade through the braid, highlighting natural texture.

Crown Braid: The natural volume of wavy hair helps create a thicker, more dramatic crown braid.

3. Braiding Curly Hair

Characteristics:

- Defined curls: Curly hair has a well-defined curl pattern, making it naturally voluminous and bouncy.
- Prone to tangles: Curly hair can easily tangle, which may make sectioning and braiding more challenging.
- Prone to dryness: Curly hair tends to be drier than straight or wavy hair, so moisture retention is key.

Braiding Techniques:

- Detangle Before Braiding: Use a wide-tooth comb or your fingers to gently detangle the hair before braiding. This ensures smooth, clean sections.

- Moisturize for Definition: Apply a curl cream, leave-in conditioner, or lightweight oil to the hair before braiding. This helps lock in moisture and enhances the natural curl pattern, making braids look more defined.

- Protective Styles: Braids such as box braids, cornrows, or twists work particularly well for curly hair, keeping it tangle-free and protecting it from environmental damage.

- Avoid Tight Tension: Be mindful of the tension when braiding. Pulling too tightly on curly hair can cause breakage, especially at the roots. Opt for looser braids that still hold the curl definition but don't tug at the scalp.

Best Styles:

- Box Braids: Ideal for protecting curly hair while offering a long-lasting, low-maintenance style.
- Dutch Braids: The underhand technique of a Dutch braid adds texture and volume to already voluminous curly hair.
- Goddess Braids: A more oversized, statement-making braid that highlights the natural texture and volume of curly hair.

4. Braiding Coily/Kinky Hair (Type 4 Hair)

Characteristics:

- Tight coils or kinks: Coily hair has a dense curl pattern that often shrinks significantly in length.
- Highly voluminous: Coily hair naturally has a lot of body and volume.

- Prone to dryness and breakage: Coily hair is more fragile, requiring extra moisture and care to avoid breakage during styling.

Braiding Techniques:

- Stretch the Hair Before Braiding: Coily hair tends to shrink, so stretching the hair by blow-drying on a low heat setting or using the banding method helps elongate the strands for easier braiding.

- Deep Condition: Always moisturize the hair before braiding. Use a rich leave-in conditioner or oil to seal in moisture and prevent the hair from drying out while in braids.

- Protective Styles: Box braids, knotless braids, Senegalese twists, and cornrows are popular styles for coily hair because they protect the hair while keeping it tucked away and out of the elements.

- Gentle Tension: Avoid braiding too tightly, especially around the edges and hairline. Coily hair is more susceptible to traction alopecia (hair loss due to tension), so it's essential to be gentle while braiding.

Best Styles:

- Knotless Box Braids: These are a protective style that puts less tension on the scalp compared to traditional box braids, making them ideal for coily hair.
- Cornrows: A classic protective style that can be worn in various patterns and sizes, offering versatility.
- Two-Strand Twists: These twists are a great low-tension alternative to braids, allowing for easy maintenance while protecting the hair.

Tips for All Hair Types

Avoid Tight Braids: No matter your hair type, avoid pulling the hair too tightly when braiding, as it can lead to scalp discomfort, tension headaches, and even hair loss.

Use a Satin or Silk Scarf: To maintain braids overnight and reduce frizz, wrap your braids in a satin or silk scarf, or sleep on a satin pillowcase.

Keep the Scalp Moisturized: Especially with protective styles like box braids or cornrows, keeping the scalp hydrated is essential. Use lightweight oils like jojoba or argan oil to keep the scalp healthy without causing buildup.

Finish with Hairspray or Serum: For extra hold, use a light mist of hairspray to set the braids in place. A shine serum can also be applied to give the braids a sleek, polished finish.

Note: Braiding is versatile and can be adapted to all hair types and textures. Whether you have fine, wavy, curly, or coily hair, there are specific techniques and styles that will enhance your natural hair texture while providing structure, elegance, and protection. By understanding your hair's unique characteristics, you can choose the right products, braiding techniques, and styles to achieve beautiful, long-lasting braids.

Conclusively: When it comes to perfecting hair braiding, patience and practice are your best allies. Whether you're just starting or looking to refine your skills, remember that every twist, turn, and braid brings you closer to perfecting your craft.

So keep pushing forward, trust your hands, and soon enough, you'll braid with confidence and finesse.

www.ingramcontent.com/pod-product-compliance
Lightning Source LLC
Chambersburg PA
CBHW051605250726
48653CB00004BA/1343